Roger Dyson, a qualified teacher with the General Council and Register of Consultant Herbalists and then went on to study at the College of Homœopathy, graduating in 1983.

As a registered member of the Society of Homœopaths and Fellow of the Register of Herbalists he practices in South East London, lectures at various colleges and holds seminars around the country.

Roger lives in Sydenham with his wife Judy. His interests include performing as an American square dance and barn dance caller, canoeing and sailing with his two children James and Charles.

Jean Cole is a registered homœopath who graduated from the College of Homœopathy in 1989. In addition to her interest in homœopathy she has also qualified in bio-mobility and spinal touch and is a registered allergy therapist using applied kineisiology

She has practises in both South East London and Sevenoaks where she lives with her three teenage children.

Jean Cole and Roger Dyson practice at the Newlands Park Natural Heath Centre, 48 Newlands Park, Sydenham, London SE26 5NE Tel: 0181 659 5001.

Comments and queries about this book may be made in writing direct to the authors at the above address or through Winter Press.

Classical Homœopathy Revisited

by
Jean Cole LCH, UKHMA
&
Roger Dyson FRH, MCH, RSHom

Winter Press
16 Stambourne Way
West Wickham
Kent BR4 9NF

First published by Winter Press in 1997
Reprinted 2000

ISBN 1 874581 04 5

Cover design by Peter and Colin Winter

Printed by Biddles of Guildford, Surrey

This book is presented as a collection of natural remedies
and as an aid in understanding their use. It is intended
for use by professional homœopaths and not as a
replacement for professional consultation or treatment.

CONTENTS

DEDICATION

This book is dedicated to the memory of
Pritam Singh Ghattaoraya, who showed us
the key to the classical texts and charged us
with the task of passing on the relevance of
the classical writers to the modern world.

FOREWORD

BY ROBERT DAVIDSON

In a time where everything is changing faster than we can imagine, homœopathy seems to be in danger of becoming stuck. In a time where the kinds and quantities of human illness are changing beyond our worst nightmares, homœopathy has to be ruthlessly realistic simply in order to meet the coming challenges of the 21st century. In a time where the old and trusted forms of things are breaking down, or being changed beyond recognition, simple similarity seems to be in some kind of danger. There seems to be currently two main streams of response in the homœopathic community to the uncertainty and changeability of our times.

The first response is to cling fanatically to the forms of the past, and be righteous and superior to other homœopaths with different approaches. This is shown at its most excessive by some followers of so called 'classical homœopathy'. These rigid and prejudiced practitioners are the exponents of merely one of homœopathy's many art forms. In fact, throughout the whole two hundred year history of homœopathy, the strictly 'classical' practitioners were always a very small minority, but were unfortunately often the fanatics who wrote most of the theoretical books. To my mind, their case is not helped by the evidence of history, which shows that it is hardly ever possible to solve the healing problems of today with the methods of the past.

The second response is to dilute and damage homœopathy with all sorts of other unnecessary filters and interpretation devices. These currently include the following: psychotherapy, allopathy, astrology, pseudo-scientific ideas, various mysticisms, psychic interpretations, etc, etc. These ideas and beliefs merely complicate and filter a simple direct perception of 'what is to be cured', without adding anything to the clarity and directness. This tends to make the 'esoteric practitioners' internal world more important than the patients' health. Genuine curative results become subservient to the perceived truth.

What I write above does not mean that I devalue or necessarily reject any of these other 'ideological intrusions' into homœopathy, but they need to be in their own place, where their true usefulness can be developed, away from homœopathy, which does not need them. To my mind, all these psychological, psychic and pseudo-spiritual distractions are being applied with over-enthusiastic naivity, and are distracting many practitioners away from the elegance of the 'simple similarity' of homœopathy.

In my opinion, the goal of homœopathy is not to be 'right', or glamorous, or spiritual; it is not to be acceptable to the establishment; it is not to become an academic qualification; the high goal of homœopathy is to be continuously useful in healing the sick in the simplest, fastest, easiest and most harmless way possible, (does this sound familiar?).

Simple homœopathy, in the hands of Hahnemann and his pupils, showed fierce and continuous development. From my perspective, homœopathy has hardly started on its journey of miracles, and it is almost a crime to crystallise the ideas, developmental approaches and practical techniques that feed the wide and hopeful future possibilities of homœopathy. Homœopathy is really a thousand year art only two hundred years young.

So what is homœopathy? It is the simple task of seeing the

patient just the way they are, right now, and finding the matching symptom picture in the materia medica. In these times, the symptom picture can actually be quite complex to match and may involve more than one remedy and more than one dose. We homœopaths owe it to our patients to continue to be simple and practical in our ideas, our approach and especially in our teaching and encouragement of the homœopaths of the future.

Much is spoken and written in homœopathy about how to interpret what Hahnemann wrote. If we look at what he consistently demonstrated throughout his life, in his actions, it becomes very simple:

1 Have no beliefs or limiting ideas.
2 Do what works best, right now.
3 Continue looking for what works better.

The true inheritors of this living torch of homœopathy should be proud to describe themselves as disciples of the ruthless practicality with which Samuel Hahnemann lived homœopathy. This means concentrating on a simple thing called results. The only good result for a homœopath is a cured patient. There are no points to be had for doing it the 'right way', or the most 'fashionable way', or the 'esoteric way', if it does not result in a cured patient. This is especially pertinent if applying 'the law of similars' in a different method may have produced the cure, and yet the patient was sacrificed to the practitioner's narrowness of mind.

A problem I have met many times is the person who has learned only one way of practising, and condemns his patient to the limitations of that one 'right'way. If the patient does not get better then it must either be the patient's fault, or the practitioners fault (the right remedy was not found). In almost every such case, a different way of applying the idea of similars, ie using a different method of practice, would have produced a different and probably much better result. However, those who know 'the truth' are not readily teachable.

The book you are about to read is unlike any other recent homœopathic book. It is filled with strange new ideas such as descending the potencies, repeating the remedies frequently, using a multiplicity of nosodes and more. Many of the rules placed on homœopathy by J.T. Kent, in his attempt to make homœopathy fit his religious and metaphysical belief structures, are left in ruins by page 50. The very interesting fact is that all of the techniques described in the book can be justified by reference to 'classical' homœopathic textbooks, as the authors clearly point out.

The issues of method and style should not be underestimated, since they are based on how we look at 'what is to be cured'. Over the last 25 years of observing and treating patients, it is obvious that patients have changed dramatically in that time, certainly for those of us practising in cities such as London. The simple, direct, 'totality' remedy, which used to work so well in about 70% of patients in 1974, is now presenting in only about 30% of patients. I thought for some years that it was my own limitation; that I just couldn't see the totalities presenting. However, prolonged consulatation and conversation with many practitioners over the last ten years has confirmed that the nature of patients has radically changed. They are more suppressed, more organically damaged, lack recuperative energy and worst of all they seem to be dis-integrating. The 'whatever it is'that holds them together as a singular functioning totality, is finally starting to break down. This presents us with patients who seem to carry all of their past traumas, injuries, poisonings and conditions with them into the present; patients who seem to have split into separate pieces each of which can have a remedy picture, a dyscrasia, an aetiology, an associated dysfunctional organ, etc.

The massive increase in sub-nutrition, the omnipresent pollution and well-intentioned allopathic poisoning (such as vaccinations, antibiotics, steroids and hormones), are doubtless the main factors responsible for this steady decline in human health. This makes it a necessity and a duty of all homœopaths to keep exploring the boundaries of their technology, just to keep up with the ever-increasing pace with which our potential patients are deteriorating.

In recent years, several very valuable methods of practice have been developed, including the 'layers' method of Eizayaga, the 'sequential prescribing' method of Lisa Monk, and with this book, the 'miasmatic' method of Pritam Singh. Hopefully, a more widespread appreciation of this range of invaluable methods of practice will come out of publications such as this; I certainly hope so.

I heartily and mindily endorse this book. It contains a description of a method of practice at first appearance quite complicated in its application, yet simple in its perception of 'what is to be cured'. I congratulate both authors on their courage to write and publish a book covering such a controversial and under-explored area of homœopathy; as if a technical homœopathy book was not unusual enough.

The method of practice outlined in this book works, it works really well. It deserves your study and responsible experiment. If you have reached this far, then I thank you, and encourage you to read the book which follows with an open mind and heart, being willing to find what is of value. All your present and future patients will be thankful for your persistance of curiosity and your integrity as a healer.

Anyone wishing to respond to this foreword, for which the authors bear no responsibility other than asking me to write one, could send comments to my Email address given below. I would prefer if people did not react from theory or prejudice, but tried the method out in practice and then responded from their experience.

Robert Davidson, June 1997

Principal, The College of Practical Homœopathy (UK).
Telephone: (44) 07000-777-654
Email: Prachom@this.is
Website: http://www.learnhomoeopathy.com

INTRODUCTION

REDISCOVERING HAHNEMANN

It was 5.30 am on the M1 and we were on our way to Leicester again. Sleepy but full of anticipation - what would we discover on this visit? We had been doing this every six weeks for the past year and had learnt much. We were two traditionally trained homœopaths who had first heard of Pritam Singh through a colleague, we had been intrigued by what we had heard, contacted him and been invited to hear more.

Our first visit challenged all our preconceptions of homœopathy and sent us scurrying to re-read or in some cases read for the first time, some of the works of the early homœopathic writers. Pritam Singh knew, "The Organon" word for word, he knew all Kent's writings inside out, he would quote verbatim, to prove a point, items from Hahnemann's "Chronic Diseases". Clarke, Nash, Allen were all familiar to him. He was in short thoroughly conversant with all the major writers of homœopathy. He had studied science in all its forms and in addition to all this he had a grounding in Ayuvedic medicine.

From all this knowledge he had developed a new perspective of homœopathy and had incorporated it in a method of treatment for twentieth century diseases and health problems, yet soundly based on the original concepts.

Much of what we learnt is in the following chapters. Information that can be found in the early writings but which has been ignored or not given much credence to in the search for the similimum. We will show that there are many considerations that can be made to enable homœopathic remedies to work reliably and repeatedly to bring about effective results in the majority of cases.

First we go back to the beginnings. Samuel Hahnemann published his first edition of "The Organon of Medicine" in 1810, in which he set out the basic principles of homœopathy that he had been working on for the previous twenty years and which still apply to this day. He stated quite simply that disease is an alteration of the inner workings of the human organism and the only visible sign of this is the observable symptoms of illness. The totality of these symptoms is the outward manifestation of the inner disease. He then stated that if these symptoms are matched with a substance that causes similar symptoms in a healthy body then cure will result. These were the basic principles used by Kent and all the early homœopaths who had no access to his later writings and the principles that the majority of present day homœopaths use.

However, Hahnemann, like present day homœopaths, found that this was not necessarily enough to obtain a complete cure and went on to experiment and develop his methods in the search for better results. To this end he developed his theory of miasms saying that disease was a manifestation of inherited taints - the miasms, and that these must be dealt with before a cure could be possible. He also mentioned the acquired taints or dyscrasias, such as mercury from allopathic (orthodox) medicines of the time and how that could affect health and could even cause a blockage in the ability of homœopathic remedies to cure. These miasms and dyscrasias are as relevant today as they were in Hahnemann's day, if not more so. Orthodox medical research is coming to the realisation that many diseases seem to have a genetic link or at least that we are born with a genetic predisposition for certain diseases.

Also there are many more toxic substances present now than in Hahnemanns's day, which we come into unavoidable contact with every day that affect our health in a subtle or even not so subtle way. The miasm theory has been given lip service in the majority of prescribing with the odd nosode being given when we do not know what else to give, (a nosode being a remedy made from any disease product). The miasmatic and dyscrasia remedies need to be given to effect a lasting cure and part of this book details how this can be done.

On re-reading Kent we noticed that he had a lot to say in many of his lectures about the depth of action of remedies. He had experience of some remedies causing aggravations because they were deep acting and if given too soon in a case could cause unnecessary suffering or did not work at all. This too needs to be taken into account in our present day prescriptions and we have included a chapter on how this can be considered.

There are many other considerations that can be made when prescribing to enable the indicated remedy to do its work effectively: considerations that were addressed by the early homœopaths but which have been disregarded as time has gone by. Techniques such as drainage and support of certain organs while the healing process is continuing. Information can also be gleaned from these early publications on how to get the best results from our polycrest remedies, bearing in mind that Hahnemann only used about thirty remedies and achieved a successful practice. Polycrest remedies being those commonly prescribed remedies covering a wide range of symptoms.

And what about potency? We now realise that each potency has a different potential for healing and when a person displays symptoms of a particular remedy he will need it in all its field of action to get the best results. Hahnemann also had something to say on mental illness and indeed displayed an understanding far in advance of the lunatic asylums that were present in his day. But when should we prescribe on the mental symptoms and when should the physical symptoms take precedence? This again is addressed in a later chapter.

"The controversy between the orthodox and modern homœopath is futile, neither of them can deliver the goods as both are extremists and therefore devoid of balance and insight. The orthodox is lost in the past and the modern homœopath is blind with the latest glitters of scientific discoveries" - K.N. Mathew MBBS, MF Hom, 1971, in his Foreword to "Radium as an Internal Remedy" by John Clarke MD.

What was written 25 years ago is even more true today. We have practitioners calling themselves 'Classical Homœopaths' promulgating a way of prescribing which the classical exponents like Hahnemann and Kent had abandoned because of its slow and at times suppressive nature. We also have a new wave of modernist homœopaths using pseudo-scientific equipment and more and more bizarre remedies. We have endeavoured in this book to bring classical homœopathy up to date and to enable the practitioner or student of average competence to achieve results which they thought impossible without another 20 years of hard study behind them.

Hahnemann had a mind far ahead of his time and like all such people met with much criticism. His work "Chronic Diseases" was regarded by some of his fellow homœopaths as the ramblings of an old man. He was well aware of the criticisms and realised he would not be understood by his contemporaries and in his preface he wrote, "A more conscientious and intelligent posterity will alone have the advantage to be obtained by a faithful punctual observance of the teachings here laid down".

This book is based very much on what we learnt from Pritam Singh tempered with our own experience. Hopefully all of us are the, "more conscientious and intelligent posterity" that Hahnemann spoke of and can learn from "faithful observation" of his writings and others like him to bring homœopathy into the modern world.

CHAPTER ONE

MIASM - FACT OR FANTASY?

It is common for practitioners to pay lip service to the existence of
the miasms. The philosophy of them is taught in the various colleges where homœopaths are trained and yet often little is taught
or understood about their practical application in prescribing.
Even Dr Herring in his introductory remarks to the third edition of
"The Organon" wrote, "What important influence can it exert
whether a homœopath adopt the theoretical opinions of
Hahneman or not, so long as he holds the principal tools of the
master and the materia medica of our schools? What influence can
it have, whether a physician adopt or reject the psoric theory, so
long as he always selects the most similar medicine possible?".
Allen replies to this in "The Chronic Miasms" that such knowledge
is, "the difference between an intelligent warfare and fighting in
the dark" as what we can see and hear from our patients is only
about some, "small fragment of a deep seated disease". According
to Hahnemann we will not get the true similimum without prescribing the nosodes and deep seated miasmatic remedies.

PSORIC MIASM

Hahnemann published six editions of his work on homœopathic philosophy - "The Organon" - the last edition being around 1834. The three later editions all incorporated considerable advances in thought and these were amplified in his book "Chronic Diseases".

Samuel Hahnemann was concerned that the way he had been previously prescribing was suppressive and too slow in obtaining results and he began to experiment with the frequent repetition and alternation of remedies, with using descending potencies and with the miasms. His use of the LM potencies came later.

Unfortunately his ideas about the miasms (literally meaning a noxious swamp) were not properly understood, so that many of his disciples denounced him and so it came into folk lore that he was getting old, senile and lazy. But as Rima Handley wrote in "A Homœopathic Love Story", "What was the miasm theory other than an early attempt to explain why some very virulent infections are not annihilated by any drugs or treatments but only change their form or site of expression?".

Why was he thought of as being lazy? Homœopaths today can spend a long time with a patient working out the first remedy. Sometimes they will send the patient home with a promise to post the medicine on after spending time pouring through books and interrogating the diagnostic computer to compare possible remedies. Hahnememann began to start nearly all his chronic cases with *Sulphur*, emphasising not the differences between them, but rather the common ground.

Hahnemann begins "Chronic Diseases" by saying that it was written after he had gained experience and he then goes on to confess the difficulties which he had experienced up to that time in curing deep seated conditions despite the ever growing number of medicines at his command.

He wrote that numerous circumstances often caused conditions which had been homœopathically overcome to rear their heads again often with changed symptomatology. The symptoms would be equally or more obstinate and troublesome as before and would take the homœopath back to his books looking for another medicine. This would be given again and once again the patient would be in a better state for a while. However the more often this happened - and happen it did with shorter periods of respite - the less effective became the remedies regardless of potency and repetition. In the end they were hardly working as weak palliatives and the disease process continued unabated with the patient getting worse from year to year.

Hahnemann's indictment of what is often considered to be classical prescribing was that from a promising beginning the progress became less favourable and the outcome hopeless. Much time was spent by Hahanemann considering the reasons for this. He concluded that the answer was not as he had written previously that the symptoms of the patient were the only thing needing to be treated, but rather that the symptoms represented a small fragment of a deep seated disease.

This disease he labelled 'psora'; the disease of suppression, deficiency and malassimilation. He had seen the continual allopathic suppression of external skin complaints with sulphur and mercury, and had seen deterioration in people's health after this had happened. He knew how the body tried to eliminate toxins, how the skin was the largest eliminative organ of the body and how people had tried to suppress itching skin eruptions from earliest times. When talking to patients who had been slow to respond he would often find this "original itch eruption". Nash took this into account when he wrote in his materia medica, "Psorinum is also found useful in the consequences of suppressed eruptions and in such cases should never be forgotten....". ("Leaders" p289). The nutrition diseases and functional disorders together with deficiency diseases were all embraced in this great classification of disease. In this respect a cause of psora is seen as the inability of the body to assimilate the complete range of nutrients required for its preservation of health or the lack of these nutrients in the diet over a long period of time. The inability of the body to assimilate the various nutrients which are so essential to its health is in part due to emotional stresses and strains which in their turn produce the functional disorders which themselves are largely responsible for the non-assimilation of nutrient factors occurring often in such small quantities and yet without which life cannot survive.

Hahnemann wrote that gradually he discovered a better way of treating this condition, and chose to start the majority of his cases with *Sulphur* - his leading anti-psoric remedy to deal with this suppression. As a sulphurous volcano will erupt from the inside, so the body will try to eliminate toxins outwards causing a myriad of skin eruptions - all these are covered by the symptomatology of *Sulphur* as a remedy.

Today with the toxicity of our bodies, *Sulphur* can react quite violently in skin conditions especially, and often the remedy *Psorinum*, the nosode from scabies, can be used instead, just as effectively but with a milder action. Scabies was extremely common in Hahnemann's day but it should be noted that scabies was used as an umbrella term for skin diseases in much the same way that leprosy was used in Biblical translations.

Sulphur is not the answer to cure everyone's ills. It does however have what Catherine Coulter describes as the, "tug-boat role" of the nosodes in that it prepares the way for the similium to work more effectively and profoundly. ("Portraits of Homœopathic Medicines", C. Coulter)

According to Hahnemann the cure of the psoric conditions can never be accomplished with *Sulphur* alone ("Chronic Diseases", p105), a fact testified to by homœopaths despite the strong indications for the remedy. It will stimulate vitality and start the healing process. However Hahnemann goes on to say that chronic diseases are seldom cured by a single remedy but require several remedies, "in the worst case the use of quite a number of them - one after the other, for its perfect cure". If we needed several remedies in succession for the worst cases in Hahnemann's day, how much more today when our bodies have to surmount obstacles of pollution in the atmosphere and in our food, the effects of heavy drugging, vaccinations, teeth fillings and radiation in increasing amounts?

SYCOTIC MIASM

We now turn our attention to deal with 'sycosis', which was the word Hahnemann has used to describe the constitutional effects of gonorrhoea. The word sycosis is from the Greek word meaning fig and so sycosis can alternatively be referred to as 'fig wart disease'.

From the outset we must be very clear that sycosis is not gonorrhoea. Gonorrhoea is an acute contagious disease affected by the gonococcus which takes between five and ten days for incubation. At the end of this time the acute symptoms are manifest which, if completely cured, will never lead to the development of sycosis.

If, however, the acute stage of the disease is badly treated and the symptoms suppressed, it will then become a systemic stigma gradually involving every life cell of the organism and in this stage it can be passed from mother to child with destructive and tragic results.

The first symptoms of sycosis after suppression are often anaemia with general chronic catarrhal conditions and invariably accompanied by inflammation of the joints and muscles and lymphatic glands. Later, such diseases as Bright's, diabetes and even cancerous conditions of the breast and uterus in the female and of the prostate in the male may ensue. Usually the patient will be completely unaware of any acute venereal disease in the family history and yet we can perceive the sycotic taints of over production, excessive discharges and hyper-function.

Samuel Hahnemann was concerned with many health problems which he saw as resulting from the constitutional effects of gonorrhoea. This was a disease which was widespread and led to catarrh, effusions, growths, warts, etc. All such similar states of over function, overproduction and hyperactivity Hahnemann classed as being part of the sycotic miasm.

Some homœopathic practitioners over the years have made life very difficult for themselves by always trying to find a specific specialised remedy for the patient. However, Hahnemann made our lives relatively simple by saying of psora, sycosis and syphilis that, "homœopathically specific remedies for each one of these three different miasmata have in great part been discovered." Later in "Chronic Diseases" he elaborates, "The gonorrhoea dependent on the fig wart miasma, as well as the above mentioned excrescences (i.e. the whole sycosis) are cured most surely and most thoroughly through the internal use of *Thuja*, which, in this case, is homœopathic", (page 84). There is no proviso, "if the symptoms agree". Hahnemann knew that the leaves of the thuja tree could cause and, therefore, cure the inherited symptoms of sycosis.

The story goes that a gardener consulted Hahnemann for treatment, who he wrongly diagnosed at first as having gonorrhoea. Apparently the gardener had the habit of chewing the leaves of the Thuja tree while going about his work and was, therefore, producing a proving of its therapeutic effects. As he stopped chewing the plant so his condition improved.

It is no coincidence that *Thuja* is the main remedy in common use for the negative and catarrhal effects of vaccination. Whatever the measure of protection of vaccinations and there are differing views on this, there is little doubt that many cases of catarrh, warts and glue ear in children emanate from the date of a vaccination showing the sycotic connection.

Allopathic medicine has little theory and philosophy of suppression, although it is a master at suppressing the immune system. For instance often a patient will tell us that an eczema suppressed by cortisone will disappear in one area only to break out again in another. Hahnemann tells us that mercury was often used by allopaths for the external destruction of sycosis, "similar excrescences then break out in other parts", (page 84).

If we go back to Hahnemann's paragraph about the use of *Thuja* we see that he says after the administration of *Thuja, Nitric acid* in potency should be used and alternated with the *Thuja* (page 84). *Nitric acid* is a mineral based remedy and therefore one which works deeper and continues the action of *Thuja*.

Nash in his "Leaders in Homœopathic Therapeutics", (page 247), wrote, "*Nitric acid* is one of our most effective antidotes to the effects of allopathic dosing with mercury in syphilis. For the other bad effects of the abuse of mercury other remedies are better, notably *Hepar sulph, Calc carb*". *Nitric acid* is, therefore, working more deeply helping to deal with any mercurial discrasia and helping not only with warts and sycotic manifestations which the *Thuja* has left behind, but also dealing with certain destructive syphilitic tendencies which need addressing.

Another remedy which is often used today instead of *Nitric acid* is *Natrum sulph*, the mineral sodium sulphate. This is another remedy complementary to and deeper than *Thuja* in its action. It does not share such deep syphilitic tendencies but has catarrh as one of its pre-eminent features and will often deal with sinus problems left behind by *Thuja*.

The Greek homœopath, George Vithoulkas, has spoken against using *Thuja* in fibroids in single doses in high potency as the stimulus can cause an enlargement of the fibroids. The writers have invariably used *Thuja* for fibroids but always in descending potencies over a period of days. This way the body is able to deal gently and gradually with the problem and the symptoms of fibroids and often the growths themselves have been found to diminish.

So when we come across a predominantly sycotic case should we start with *Thuja*? Not according to Hahnemann, as all chronic disease comes from a predominantly psoric base. ("The Organon", para 80) which is the "fundamental cause".

Hahnemann states, "it is necessary first to come to the assistance of the most afflicted part, the psora, with the specific antipsoric remedies given...., and then to make use of the remedies for sycosis." ("Chronic Diseases", page 85). The exception which we have found, is in acute sycotic conditions where giving *Psorinum* or *Sulphur* at frequent intervals does not always work but *Thuja* will produce results.

Hahnemann had a restricted knowledge of the nosode *Medorrhinum* made from the gonococcus of gonorrhoea and it was left to his followers like Kent to discover the true potential of the remedy. Kent said that, "one of the many uses of this remedy is in the inherited complaints of children".

Here follow some cases as examples of how we have treated a number of patients with sycotic symptoms to the fore. These cases will need to be read in conjunction with Appendix III to understand how we actually administer the remedies.

Case 1

A typical cure in a case of glue ear, where catarrh and sinus problems are steeped in the family background might, therefore be:-

Week 1:
Day 1 and 2   *Psorinum* in descending potencies.
Days 3 - 7   *Thuja* 30 (am) *Berberis* 30 (pm). *Thuja* precedes
               Tuberculinum well and helps it work better.
               Berberis is used to assist drainage.

Week 2:   Nil

Week 3:
Days 1 and 2   *Tuberculinum* in descending potencies
Days 3 - 7   *Thuja* 30 (am) *Hydrastis* 30 (pm)

Weeks 4 and 5:   Nil

Week 6:
Days 1 and 2   *Thuja* in descending potencies
Days 3 - 7   *Thuja* 30 (am) *Kali phos* 30 (pm) - This being a
                deeper drainage remedy.

Weeks 7,8 & 9: Nil

Week 10:
Days 1 and 2   *Medorrhinum* in descending potencies.
Days 3 - 7   *Medorrhinum* 30 (8am) *Kali phos* 30 (2pm)
                Pulsatilla 30 (8pm)

As and if necessary, we could progress with deeper drainage remedies using *Kali phos* and then *Causticum* in a variety of potencies. Alternatively we could progress to the deeper sycotic remedies of *Natrum sulph* or *Nitric acid* and then *Thuja* again. Or we could go to the syphilitic remedies, or to maximise the remedies used we could use them again in descending potencies on a daily basis.

The following are further examples of treating patients with sycotic symptoms to the fore.

Case 2
Sinusitis and Catarrh Case: Man born September 1943. Relations had sinus problems, catarrh, asthma, throat problems, arthritis and emphysema.
30.9.92 Sinusitis. Mucus trickles down the throat. Pressure in the ears. Allergic reaction has built up tissue in the ear now causing ear ache. History of bad hay fever. Stress<. Fillings ++.

Remedies given sequentially in descending order at daily intervals - *Psorinum, Hepar sulph, Thuja, Rhus tox, Tuberculinum.*
8.11.92 Much better for the first week or so, then flu which went to throat and sinuses, but sinuses not as bad as would

24

have normally expected. Sinus problems and ears ringing for last three days.
Remedies given in the same way as before - *Psorinum, Hepar sulph, Thuja,. Rhus tox and Tuberculinum.*

15.12.92 Was better immediately and generally had felt much better. Only one sinus headache. Ears less noisy. A little mucous trickles down throat.
Remedies given in the same way - *Lycopodium, Medorrhinum* and *Silica.*

16.1.93 Fine - no remedies given.

Case 3
Endometriosis Case: Woman born May 1967. Grandparents and parents had kidney problems and mother was on drugs for such problems before conception. Mother, sister and two cousins had painful periods.

24.2.93 Patient had ovarian cyst removed and endometriosis started after the operation. Periods are now always heavy with intermittent bleeding. More painful at ovulation and period time. All periods are equally bad. Tiredness, backache, Pre-menstrual tension and fluid retention with periods.
Remedies given sequentially in descending order daily - *Psorinum, Hepar sulph, Thuja* and *Sepia.*

30.3.93 "On top of the world". Period shorter than normal and more normal period pain. No tiredness. Back to old self. Premenstrual tension (PMT) lasted a day instead of a week.
Remedies given as before - *Psorinum, Hepar sulph, Thuja, Sepia* and *Tuberculinum.*

4.5.93 Period a better colour. Felt healthier. Period heavy but for a short time. Not painful at ovulation. Said, "It is the difference between existing and living". Craves sweet things less. All pain is less intense and less frequent. Not taken a paracetamol since started treatment. More energy. No remedies given.

14.9.93 A few stress headaches. Feels better within self. Ovulation pain shorter.
Remedies given:
Days 1 and 2   *Psorinum*
Days 3 - 7   *Hepar sulph* 30 (8am), *Nux vomica* 30 (2pm), *Sepia* 30 (8pm)
Gurnsey mentions how *Nux vomica* is able to precede *Sepia*

25

and increase its effectiveness.

10.11.93 Periods fine and energy good. Experienced pain for eight days with the stress and emotions involved in a relationship break-up.

Days 1 and 2   *Psorinum*

Days 3 - 7   *Hepar sulph* 30 (8am) *Nux vomica* 30 (2pm) *Sepia* 30 (8pm).

22.12.93 No ovulation pain or headaches. No period pains or PMT. Fine. No remedies given.

Case 4

Fibroid Case: Woman born February 1950. Family history of cancer, TB and heart attacks.

2.9.92 Generally continual ache with fibroids all the time in the abdomen. Heartburn for 18 months. Periods heavier and now only 14 days apart. Tired. PMT makes her very intolerant. Fillings +++. Hair loss.

Remedies given sequentially daily in descending order - *Psorinum, Hepar Sulph, Thuja, Phosphorus, Tuberculinum.*

13.10.92 No pain for one week and then returned but not so badly. Milder and sore. Heartburn rare. Last period much better and only lasted 7 days. Pain only lasted 12 hours which is "remarkable - best I can remember", Energy much improved. Co-ordination better, PMT improved. Itchiness and cramp gone. Hair loss still same.

Remedies given in same way - *Psorinum, Hepar sulph, Thuja, Medorrhinum, Phytolacca.*

10.12.92 Stomach fine. No heartburn. PMT considerably less. Fibroid ache 8/10 >. Better sustained energy. Last period much more normal.

Remedies given in the same way - *Psorinum, Hepar sulph, Thuja, Medorrhinum, Phytolacca.*

26.1.93 No pain or bleeding or any indications of having a fibroid. Hair loss improved. Periods excellent. No PMT.

Remedies given *Conium* and *Wiersbaden.*

9.4.93 Had flu but fully recovered. No problems. No remedy given.

SYPHILITIC MIASM

One of, or probably the most destructive disease around in

Hahnemann's day was that of syphilis. As opposed to the under functioning of psora and the over functioning of sycosis, we have the third great miasm characterised by its destruction and necrosis of organs, bone and tissues. Hahnemann named this the 'syphilitic' or luetic miasm.

Under this heading we would group diseases such as osteo-arthritis, osteo-porosis, sickle cell anaemia and the disease recently publicised in the press - necrotising fasciites. Few people today would make any direct link between these conditions and syphilis and any link would be very theoretical and speculative. However, it can be argued that suppression of syphilis in one generation can mutate the miasm into another destructive disease in a future generation.

This was certainly the view of Kent, who said of the nosode *Syphilinum* ("Lectures on Materia Medica", p932), "Whenever the symptoms that are representative of the patient himself have been suppressed in any case of syphilis and nothing remains but weakness and a few results of the storm that has long ago or recently passed, this nosode will cause reaction and restore order and sometimes do much curing...."

There have been many theories as to the origin of syphilis, but there is considerable doubt as to the accuracy of any of the theories. It is certain that this disease struck Europe towards the end of the fifteenth century when 'pestilence' of all kinds appeared on this continent. In 1489 there was a violent epidemic of typhus in Spain and in 1492 a diphtheria epidemic struck Germany followed swiftly by smallpox and measles. The black date for syphilis was 1495 when it struck in Naples. The condition became more widespread in Europe during the fifteenth and sixteenth centuries, spread in part by vast movements of troops and soldiers. The more people travelled, the more the disease spread.

It was severe and loathsome in its symptoms. The skin rotted in leprous like patches, ulcers festered and destroyed flesh and bone. Eruptions gnawed the mouth, throat, nose and eyes. The sex organs were particularly affected. Physicians applied mercurial preparation in an effort to get rid of all these dreadful symptoms. Compounds of sulphur, guaiacum and a multitude of others were all useless. Rapidly syphilis saturated the continent of Europe and entered Asia and Africa.

The 'best' doctors were those who could most quickly suppress the symptoms. In 1725 Cromwell's army invaded Scotland and Sibbens (means wild strawberries) appears on the scene. This disease resembled tropical syphilis or Yaws (also known as framboise - raspberries, or pian - strawberries). It began with bright red protruding ulcers like raspberries, progressing to the destruction of the mouth and throat. Like all syphilis, it was transferred by contact during sexual intercourse. Yaws and Sibbens were related but how it migrated from Africa to Scotland in those days no one knows.

The World Health Organisation has conducted an examination of eight million people in Haiti, Indonesia, Thailand and the Philippines and of these two million were found to be infected with yaws. A quarter of a million Mexicans are known to suffer from pinta, carate or quirico and in 1938 it was classified as a syphilitic disease perpetuated by the same methods. Here is the proof of how widespread this disease became and how with its insidious progress from generation to generation, it has become so deeply ingrained in the constitutions of the peoples of this planet. A taint indeed and one that in contradiction to the overgrowth of tissue which is characteristic in sycosis, is easily diagnosed by its destructive effect on tissue.

Syphilis invades the body through minute breaks in the skin or mucous membranes and the period of incubation is from four to six weeks, during which time the victim is completely unaware of any symptoms. Then appears a bright red ulcer, usually about one centimetre in diameter, at the site of contagion which in some circumstances will grow to a larger size. Without any treatment at all this ulcer will heal. This is known as the soft chancre and is the first stage of syphilis.

The second stage usually commences about one month after the first stage, but may appear as late as three months after the ulcer. It may be pointed out that the ulcer at the site of contagion is usually to be found either on the genital organs of male or female or on the lips. The second stage is characterised by headaches without apparent cause, coming and going at intervals, periodic fevers with skin rashes which may take the form of any known skin disease. These skin rashes will heal and for a time disappear, only to recur at intervals. The headaches are usually worse at night. Another feature of this stage is pains in the joints and bones and there may be severe anaemia. It is during this stage that it penetrates the nervous system although there may by no symptoms at all of nervous disease. In this stage too the walls of the blood vessels, the heart and other organs of the body are penetrated. Left untreated this stage too will clear up and the symptoms disappear. There is then a period of freedom which may last from two to twenty years, after which the onset of the third stage will occur.

There is no organ or part of the body which may not be attacked during the third stage of syphilis. Generally this takes the form of tumour like masses which become soft in the centre and ulcerate. These masses are called gummas and the resultant ulcers are extremely difficult to heal. These ulcers can occur in the skin, bones, joints, liver and also the palate, mouth and tongue. Disease will also occur of the large blood vessels and later the germs which have settles in the brain and spinal cord and remained undestroyed will give rise to disease of the nervous system such as locomotor ataxia and general paralysis of the insane.

Many suppressive drugs and compounds have at various times during the history of syphilis been hailed as miracles and certain cures. Many of these will destroy the germ of syphilis while others only partially so. All will leave a miasm or taint in the organs. The spirochete is now proclaimed resistant in some of its strains to the latest antibiotic treatment.

Hahnemann stated that syphilis is a chronic disease. He uses the word "chronic" in the sense of miasms which he applies whether the manifestations are acute or long lasting. The difference between the acute and chronic diseases is that in the acute there is complete recovery or death. In the chronic miasms, the conditions continue in varying degrees throughout life. Hahnemann states that a cure can be effected by the correctly chosen remedy. This has been proven time and time again. The correct homœopathic remedy will always stimulate the body's energy system to bring about a cure unless the pathology has progressed too far. We are concerned here with the effects upon the offspring of a syphilitic union which will not show the primary ulcer. The disease in this case has been welded into the very fibre of the child's being.

Whatever the historical facts, we know that in such

29

syphilitic remedies as *Mercurius, Syphilinum* and *Fluoric acid* we have medicine to help in a large number of cases of destructive pathology. The majority of our syphilitic remedies come from mineral sources which have a slower pace of action than many of our medicines made from plants. Cases where the syphilitic miasm is predominant, therefore, will not be resolved as rapidly as cases involving mainly the sycotic or functional psoric miasms. However, by following the guidelines laid down by Samuel Hahnemann we can treat cases with confidence and know that we will get results as far as the patients vitality is capable of achieving those results.

Kent, as a result of experience, knew that latent syphilis, or a latent destructive tendency would often exist in a patient where it was least expected. He also knew that when anti-psoric remedies were continually used in high potency, the under functioning of the system could be easily turned into destructive functioning where syphilis was latent.

He wrote about this in his, "Lectures on Materia Medica" (p987), when he said that many times he had observed conditions taking on, "destructive ulcerations in old broken-down cases after *Sulphur* has been given and that *Syphilinum* will restrain it and establish repair. *Sulphur* often produces prolonged aggravations when there are many tissue changes in advanced cases of syphilis ...... The effort of *Sulphur* is to remove the results of disease which the patient cannot stand. It often causes suspicion of latent syphilis when such aggravations are very severe after *Sulphur* high. *Sulphur* low will not be followed by such results. After such prolonged aggravations *Syphilinum* should be considered. Latent syphilis often exists where it is least expected. This nosode should be used only in high potencies." The above passage may be read with more understanding if the word *Sulphur* is substituted for "an anti-psoric remedy".

This led Pritam Singh to use a single dose of *Syphilinum* in a high potency prophylactically to prevent the manifestation of latent syphilis. We have continued this practice and when using several anti-psoric remedies in descending potencies starting from high potencies it is normal for us to use on one day a single dose of *Syphilinum* in a high potency. As the action of the dose of *Syphilinum* is used up in dealing with the latent aspect, we would need to use *Syphilinum* again in a strong syphilitic case, often in a range of potencies, to deal with the miasmatic background. And as we know that, "latent syphilis often exists where it is least expected ", (Kent), there is no way that we could really anticipate which are the cases where we need to use *Syphilinum*. This leads us to use *Syphilinum* in a fairly routine manner in order to prevent any such tendency.

However, when we are dealing with a strongly syphilitic case what does Hahnemann have to teach us about methodology? He says that the first step. after paying attention to diet and life-style, is to give **anti-psoric** medicine. The syphilitic miasm is combined with the psoric and the "internal slumbering psora" has been awakened. Further anti-psoric medicine will be needed before we address the syphilitic miasm and because of the widespread allopathic suppression of syphilis by mercury, Hahnemann considered *Hepar sulph* to be preferred to pure *Sulphur* as it is antidotal to a mercurial dyscrasia.

Where there are strong symptoms of the psoric, sycotic and syphilitic miasms, again Hahnemann wrote, (p100, "Chronic Diseases"), "The psora was treated first, then one of the other two chronic miasmata, the symptoms of which were at the time the most prominent, and then the last one. The remaining psoric symptoms had then still to be combated with suitable remedies and then lastly what there yet remained of sycosis or syphilis....."

It may be that the total constitution in a case is but little changed until we have used the deeper acting syphilitic remedies.

Hahnemann illustrates this by an account of a tiler infected with venereal disease and overdosed with mercury. Anti-psoric remedies improved his ulcers and further progress was made by sycotic remedies. It then needed the syphilitic remedy of *Protoxide of Mercury* in potency to restore him virtually to full health, ("Chronic Diseases").

Sickle Cell Anaemia Case: West Indian man born March l966. Heart conditions in family background.

15.7.91 Tired. Joint pains. Picks up infections easily with his condition. Pains are worse after exertion. Pains disappear as he loosens up with gentle movement. Knee joint can be stiff. Heat improves. Cold aggravates. Has flushes of heat. A born worrier. Stress aggravates. Teeth fillings ++.

Remedies given sequentially in descending potencies daily. *Psorinum, Hepar sulph, Rhus tox, Tuberculinum.*

10.9.91 Less tired spells than usual. No joint pains. No flushes of heat. Feels better in himself. Remedies given in same way as before. *Psorinum, Hepar sulph, Thuja,. Rhus tox, Tuberculinum.*

26.11.91 Finished remedies a month ago and then in hospital for two days with a crisis and severe pains. Tiredness improved since first seen. Knee joint not stiff now but can click at times. As he works in a hospital he had polio, hepatitis and tetanus vaccinations previous week. Colour of eyes less yellow.

Remedies given as before - *Psorinum, Hepar sulph, Thuja, Ferrum phos, Syphilinum.*

4.2.92 Fine while on remedies. Two weeks later felt tired but not as much as previously. No aches, pains or stiffness. Eyes still less yellow.

Remedies given - *Psorinum, Hepar sulph, Thuja, Ferrum phos* and *Syphilinum.*

31.3.92 Generally fine. Not tired. Finished remedies 3 weeks ago. No aches, pains or stiffness. 9/10 improvement.

Remedies - *Psorinum, Hepar sulph, Ferrum phos, Medorrhinum, Carbo animalis.*

20.8.92 Fine. No remedies given.

Leg Ulcer Case: Woman age 63 with leg ulcer that appeared after a fall. Oozing slightly.

Remedies

Day 1 and 2	*Psorinum*
Days 3 - 7	*Hepar sulph 30* (8am), *Berberis 30* (2pm), *Rhus tox 30* (8pm)
Days 8 - 15	Nil

| Days 16 - 17 | *Tuberculinum* (This covers both sycotic and syphilitic and the latent psora.) |
| Days 18 - 22 | *Hepar sulph 30, Kali phos 30, Rhus tox 30* |

Following that no remedies were given for two weeks during which time the oozing stopped and the smell improved.

Then,

| Days 1 and 2 | *Kali phos* |
| Days 3 - 7 | *Kali phos 30* (8am), *Rhus tox 30* (2pm), *Hepar sulph 30* (8pm). |

No remedies for three weeks.

Then

| Days 1 and 2 | *Causticum* |
| Days 3 - 7 | *Rhus tox 30* (8am), *Causticum 30* (8pm). |

After this there was a 65% improvement and remedies were taken into depth, given in descending potencies sequentially on a daily basis - *Psorinum, Hepar sulph, Rhus tox, Syphilinum, Lycopodium, Silica* and *Carbo animalis*.

After this she was fine and no more remedies were needed.

LATENT PSORA OR THE TUBERCULAR MIASM

Tuberculosis is a specific infectious disease produced by the Mycobacterium tuberculosis or Tubercle bacillus. Most infections enter by the respiratory tract and attack the lungs but many organs can be affected. TB is a very common disease in many countries throughout the world and has been for a great many years. As a result we are all being continually exposed to infection and it is not hard to appreciate that most of us must, at one time or another, have actually been infected with the bacilli.

The initial primary infection, as it is called, usually occurs in childhood or early adult life and causes serious disease in the body only in severely debilitated and undernourished people or when the infection is extremely heavy and persistent. In most people, with good defences, no illness results from the primary infection and it probably serves to protect the patient against further attacks. Avoidance of overcrowding, bad housing and under-nutrition is of utmost importance in reducing the dangers of TB.

Just as good nutrition and hygiene can help prevent the spread of TB, so the opposite will lead to the illness which is then suppressed by drugs and driven into latency. Hahnemann spoke frequently of the suppression of psora by external factors (e.g. emotions and fatigue), intentional homœopathic suppression (see Chapter 6), unintentional homœopathic suppression as mentioned earlier (described graphically in the first few pages of "Chronic Diseases") and allopathic suppression. This suppression drives the condition into latency and many of our classical writers considered latent psora and the tubercular miasm to be one and the same.

Compton Burnett considered that patients whose parents had TB and who had inherited TB themselves were often of a feeble vitality. They were always tired, got sick easily and didn't throw off inherited tendencies. Nervousness and anaemia were common. Burnett used the remedy *Tuberculinum* in a routine way here and found that this latent susceptibility and under functioning of the system - all keynotes of psora - considerably improved. He also found considerable improvement in hyper-function and destructive pathology leading him to conclude that the tubercular miasm was not only latent psora, but by working more deeply, related to the sycotic and syphilitic miasms also.

Kent found valuable use for this remedy when his well selected remedy did not hold and when the constitution was tending to break down - a hint of its syphilitic connections. Hahnemann spoke of suppressed conditions returning to the surface in a changed format. The tubercular miasm is the miasm of change. In its provings physical symptoms change and the person has mental desires to change jobs, house, environment, social groups, etc. Seasonal conditions which change according to the time of year, such as hay fever, which spring from latency as a result of certain allergic triggers and environmental factors will often respond very effectively to *Tuberculinum*.

Perhaps we all have TB in our background if we go back far enough in the generations and Kent found the remedy very useful where there was a paucity of symptoms and some of the keynotes of tiredness and susceptibility even though he could not trace the pathology of TB.

In his lectures on *Tuberculinum*, Kent said this about the remedy: "It is deep acting, constitutionally deep, because it is a product of disease from a very deep-seated constitional condition, like *Silica* and *Sulphur*. It goes deep into the life; it is antipsoric; it is long acting, and it affects constitutions more deeply than most remedies; and when our deepest remedies act only a few weeks, and then have to be changed, this remedy comes in as one of the remedies - when the sypmtoms agree - and brings a better state of reaction, so that remedies hold longer. It may well be considered a species of *Psorinum*."

Dr James Hewlett-Parsons wrote that in the tubercular patient we find "All the mentals of predominate psora plus the destructive pathological changes of syphilis".

It is for these reasons that we usually use *Tuberculinum* as our second nosode in prescribing. We may well start with *Psorinum* (or *Sulphur*) to first attend to the more acute manifestations of the psoric miasm. After then giving unblocking and /or indicated remedies according to the symptom picture we will normally use *Tuberculinum* to deal with the latent side of psora, as well as paying attention to the other miasms. Following this we may repeat the treatment after a suitable interval, or progress to deeper acting remedies and other indicated remedies.

KENT'S VIEW OF NOSODES
Whilst we have been concerned with the development of Hahnemann, it has been considered that Kent, his eminent disciple, was working in a very different way. Certainly a reading of Kent's lectures on *Tuberculinum* would substantiate this: "I do not use *Tuberculinum* merely because it is a nosode, or with the idea that generally prevails of using nosodes; that, a product of the disease for the disease, and the result of the disease. This I fear is too much the prevailing thought in using nosodes. In certains places it prevails and is taught that anything relating to gonorrhoea must be treated with *Medorrhinum*, anything psoric must be treated with *Psorinum*, and anything that relates to tuberculosis must be treated with *Tuberculinum*. That will go out of use some day; it is mere isopathy, and it is an unsound

doctrine. It is not the better idea of Homœopathy. It is not based upon sound principles. It belongs to hysterical Homœopathy that prevails in this century. **Yet much good has come out of it.**" (Authors' emphasis)

Kent had been trained to take into account only the idea of the similimum and he developed this to produce remedy pictures or portraits. He graphically described the characteristics of the individuals who would respond to the various remedies, and developed our understanding of their mental and emotional symptomatology based on the homœopathic provings and experience. Yet due partly to the secrecy of Hahnemann himself, he did not fully understand how Hahnemann was working in the latter part of his career. Being objective he had to admit to having seen much good emanating from a routine use of the nosodes and he could see no objection based on experience, but only so far as he could not see justification based on the 'Law of Similars'. Homœopaths generally do not like the routine prescribing of specific remedies, preferring to spend time individualising often quite subjective symptoms as detailed by the patient. However, we should not be afraid of similar prescriptions as we all share such similar miasmatic backgrounds.

Later in his career Kent wrote a further book, "Clinical Cases", based on his experience and in the light of this he had obviously altered his view. He said (p511), "If you have the symptoms of *Tuberculinum*, of course you will stand by it; but in many instances .. we have nothing but the physical condition on which to depend; no symptoms. Hunt here hunt there, hunt somewhere else; you have nothing on which to depend : everything is suppression. I test such cases at once with *Tuberculinum*; or; ..... with *Psorinum*; and these tests are legitimate experiments with me." He carried on to state that he would continue with a series of potencies as the condition improved.

In Kent's "Lectures on Homœopathic Materia Medica", he noted three features in his description of remedies. Some he considered useful for specific symptomatolgy, some he described as constitutional and some he described as antipsorics.

As homœopaths prescribe on the essential elements of

pathology and personality traits, it is common for them to reach conclusions that a person is constitutionally 'Nux vomica' or 'Arsenicum album' for example

Although Kent introduced the idea of constitutional prescribing, he would disagree with these conclusions and say (under his Lecture on Sabadilla) that these are not the constitutional remedies. They are only remedies which will mitigate during severe attacks. Kent says that for example, hay fever symptoms are the outcome of the psoric constitution and such cases must be treated by anti-psorics. Only by anti-psoric remedies can the constitution be built up and with such treatment each yearly attack is lighter. Kent was thus developing, as do all researchers, in the light of experience and merging his concept of the constitutional approach into the idea of the psoric constitution and anti-psorics.

DESCENDING POTENCIES
Homœopathic medicines are commonly prescribed in a wide range of potencies or strengths. In mainland Europe, we regularly see a mixture of more than one remedy made up in the same tablet of a low potency and given 2, 3 or 4 times daily.

In this country something of a mythology has built up that the finest way to prescribe is to give a single dose of a remedy in a high strength and then to wait for a month or two or even more if necessary if the remedy appears to be working. There are indications that this is the way Hahnemann started to work; but how did he develop? What clues did his later writings and cases give us?

Hahnemann was an experimenter and wrote against any too rigid methodology. He stated that factors such as age, development, vitality, and the nature of their ailments necessitated variety in the treatment of an individual and in the way the doses were administered. In a similar way our aim in writing this book is foremostly to give the principles necessary for deriving a strategy for cure as far as the patient is capable of being cured. Our case illustrations show our methodology and therefore give guidance for formulating a framework for the principles in order that progress can be achieved.

However, Hahnemann continued that in chronic diseases he had found it best to give a dose of the medicine every one or two days, but he added that our bodies could not well bear the medicine being given in an unchanged potency. We know, however, from his own cases that he would often repeat the 30th potency and many times he alternated one remedy with another at different times of day.

As discussed elsewhere, Hahnemann would often use potencies in descending order to maximise the action of the remedy as the different potencies have a different sphere of action. Kent also wrote in his work, "Clinical Cases" that after giving *Psorinum* or *Tuberculinum* one should continue with, "a series of potencies".

Sometimes Hahneman would review progress before descending his potencies, but this was by no means the rule. He even said that with weak patients he would allow them just to smell the medicines, "but every time of a lower potency". ("Chronic Diseases", p269). We have not experimented with olfactory prescribing, but frequently we will descend our potencies from the 200, 1M or 10M, gradually building our patient up to enable the higher potencies to be taken.

MINIMUM DOSE

We would like to put here a few paragraphs about the minimum dose as it seems that from its very beginnings every aspect of homœopathy has been surrounded by controversy. Not least of these has been the idea of giving the minimum dose. Dorothy Shepherd wrote two books entitled, "Magic of the Minimum Dose" and "More Magic of the Minimum Dose". Here she said that homœopathy was based on the law of similarity and the law of potentisation. "In other words the power of the minimum dose in arresting and curing disease was proved biologically on the living organism of healthy volunteers." ("More Magic of the Minimum Dose").

Traditionally homœopaths have viewed the minimum dose as being the idea of giving one tablet of one remedy in a high potency. A close study of the classical writings, however, does bring to the fore the question; Is the minimum dose about quantity, frequency or potency?

In paragraph 60 of "The Organon", Hahnemann writes of the necessity for the allopath to give, "ever increasing quantities of the palliative" and contrasts this in his next paragraph as he writes of the need of the homœopath to give, "the most minute doses".

Arndt's Law is at the basis of all homœopathy and deals with the effect of varying doses on the vital force. Summarised it says that, 'slight stimulants quicken vitality, medium doses promote vitality, strong doses arrest it and very strong does destroy it'.

Hahnemann was well aware of these precepts when he wrote that when prescribing we give a minute dose giving only so much reaction as is necessary for the restoration of health (para 66 "The Organon"). Later he says that the suitability of a medicine does not depend on accurate homœopathic selection alone, but also on the size and smallness of the dose, and too much can be, "injurious by its mere magnitude" (para 275). He went on to say that, "Too large doses of an accurately chosen medicine especially when frequently repeated bring about much trouble as a rule". (para 276 6th Edition).

The writers have become aware of young children who had got hold of a whole bottle of their parent's tablets and taken the entire contents. The results were that they developed a proving of the remedy. This very rarely happens if just one tablet or pilule is taken. To solve the problem of what size of dose to give Hahneman recommends experiment and careful observation. ("The Organon", Para 278).

As we have said, a dose of the appropriate medicine given at 5 - 10 minute intervals will stimulate the vital force and begin to eliminate acute symptoms. We have pilules in our clinic, four of which equate in quantity to one tablet. If we give a patient one pilule at intervals of 5 minutes and after four doses the symptoms change or they feel more relaxed or better in themselves, then we know that one tablet is the optimum dose. Similarly if a patient shows no reaction until eight pilules have been taken then we know that two tablets is the optimum dose.

The more drugged a person may be with allopathic drugs the more they will need in terms of quantity. Conversely the more sensitive they are and the more they have a condition which may aggravate, the less they will need. With experience we can make a fairly accurate judgement and will not need to experiment with each new patient.

In the event that too large a dose has been given we can

divide the dose and descend the potencies more quickly. We should give only such small a dose as is needed to overpower and annihilate the disease. In this way even if the wrong medicine has been given, the body's vitality will rally to overcome any potential problem. (Para 283, "The Organon").

In case the reader still needs to be convinced as to the nature of the term 'quantity', we quote the first two sentences of para 284 of the 5th Edition of "The Organon", in its entirety which leaves us no room for doubt: "The action of a dose, moreover, does not diminish in the direct ratio of the quantity of material medicine contained in the dilutions used in homœopathic practice. Eight drops of the tincture of a medicine to the dose do not produce four times as much effect on the human body as two drops, but only about twice the effect that is produced by two drops to the dose."

CHAPTER TWO

———◦◇◦———

BARRIERS TO CURE
"THE ORGANON" PARAS 41 AND 74 REVISITED

Digestive problems are normally easily and successfully treated by homœopathic remedies so that when two friends arrived who had been recommended to see us for treatment, we had every confidence of fairly rapid improvement.

Miss F came suffering from burping, heartburn and constipation. Her symptoms had all started shortly after she had started her new job which she had found stressful. Her boss expected her to work long hours to finish the days work and to prepare for the next day. She found that when she arrived home tired, she would hurriedly bolt down a ready-made meal which would then lie heavily in her stomach for the rest of the evening. A sherry or whisky would help her to relax at the end of the day. The next day would start with two cups of coffee in order to wake her sufficiently to get into gear in order to start work.

Her symptoms, the relationship between stress and her

symptomatology and her lifestyle, all pointed towards *Nux vomica*. After *Psorinum* was given to help shift the constitutional psoric layer and to stimulate her immune system, *Nux vomica* was given daily in descending potencies with every expectation of success.

Her friend, Miss Y had also come with heartburn and bowel problems. She at times suffered from constipation and at other times from diarrhoea. All her symptoms were very changeable, were particularly brought on by the eating of rich and fatty foods and especially eggs. A walk across the park in the fresh air would make her feel better temporarily

Miss Y had started a new job at the same time as her friend. It did not appear quite as pressurised as that of Miss F, but then her capacity to cope with stress seemed lower. She would return to her husband, often quite tearful, in the evenings saying that she didn't know whether she could cope and whether she had done the right thing in taking on the job in the first place. Her symptoms were all covered by the remedy *Pulsatilla*, a plant commonly known as the meadow anemone. So for her also *Psorinum* was given daily in descending potency followed by *Pulsatilla* in the same way. Both of the above patients had a good general vitality with no serious pathological problems, and so they were safely started with the high potency of 10M to be followed by 1m, 200, 30, 12 and 6 on successive days.

The surprise came at the next consultation when neither of them had noticed any substantial improvement, although Miss Y on *Pulsatilla* had noticed a few changes. There was no doubt that the remedies were correct. They covered all the main symptoms, including the mental and emotional ones. In Hahnemann's terminology they were "in consonance" with the symptoms of the remedies. *Psorinum* had been given in its "tugboat role" of pulling through the *Nux vomica* and *Pulsatilla* and making them more effective.

There was one common link between these cases, and that was that both of the patients had become friends when they were training together as dental nurses. Their symptoms had both started when they had begun their work which involved the mixing of dental amalgam containing 50% mercury.

In Hahnemann's day he had to treat many patients suffering

from mercury poisoning which he found weakened the patient's energy. Mercury was used for biliousness, ulcers and any number of complaints in the form or calomel, corrosive sublimate and mercurial ointment. This led Hahnemann to write paragraph 74 of "The Organon" as follows: "Among chronic diseases we must unfortunately include all those widespread illnesses artificially created by allopathic treatments, by the prolonged use of violent, heroic drugs in strong increasing doses, the abuse of calomel, corrosive sublimate, mercurial ointment, nitrate of silver, iodine and its ointment, opium, valerian, cinchona bake and quinine, foxglove, Prussic acid, sulphur and sulphuric acid, perennial purgatives, bloodletting in torrents, leeches, fontanels, setons, etc.

All these relentlessly weaken the vital force and, if they do not completely exhaust it, progressively untune it, each in its own characteristic way, to such an extent that it has to bring about a revolution in the organism to maintain life against these hostile and destructive attacks. It has to inhibit or exaggerate the excitability or sensitivity of a part of the organism, dilate or contract, soften or harden or even completely destroy certain parts, and bring about internal or external lesions (internally and externally maiming the body) in order to protect the organism against complete destruction of life from the every renewed hostile attack of such ruinous forces."

He then continued in paragraph 75 and 76 to describe the difficulties in curing such patients and stressed the need for the giving of appropriate aid, "for the eradication of any chronic miasm that may happen to be lurking in the background".

So how do we go about strengthening a person with a weakened vitality and unblocking a case so affected by the inhalation of mercury. For rudimentary research showed that all the symptoms displayed by the above patients could be the effect of mercury poisoning.

One of the most well known and used books in homœopathy is "The Repertory" or dictionary of symptoms, produced from provings and clinical information compiled by James Tyler Kent and his team of doctors. On page 1374 of that book is a rubric headed, "Mercury, abuse of". This gives 47 remedies, including *Pulsatilla* which could have explained why the nurse given *Pulsatilla* appeared to have some relief. However there

are ten main remedies and the one of these which is emphasised in other writings by Kent and other writers is *Hepar sulph*,
a mineral based remedy made from a sulphate of calcium.

In his "Lectures", Kent writes, "A very important sphere
for *Hepar* is after mercurialisation. Many old people are walking the street at the present day who have been the victims of
Calomel, who have been salivated, who have taken blue pill
for recurrent bilious spells, to tap the liver...... It becomes a valuable antidote to that state of mercurialization." *Hepar sulph* is
one of our largest polycrests, (ie a commonly prescribed
remedy covering a very wide range of symptoms). It has a
multitude of digestive symptoms. *Hepar sulph* has many
symptoms related to an over sensitivity or under sensitivity of
the nervous system, and there are still many of its symptoms
of which we are not aware as it has only been proved in a
minority of potencies.

The Indian writer Bhanja in his book, "Constitution ; Drug
Pictures and Treatment" states that *Hepar sulph* should be used,
"After abuse of mercury or other metals, iodine, iodide of
potash, cod-liver oil or quinine."Hahnemann himself knew of
the value of *Hepar sulph*. He wrote of it frequently in his work,
"Chronic Diseases", and used it much in his practice. Many of
the cases that he treated, he believed had been mismanaged by
allopathic treatment with mercury and so produced symptoms
covered by the remedy *Hepar sulph*. This led him to write, "it is
nearly always necessary to give again, from time to time during
treatment, a dose of *Sulphur* or of *Hepar*...", (p128, "Chronic
Diseases"). We are also told in the same section that it is often
useful, "to interpose between the doses of pure *Sulphur*, a small
dose of *Hepar sulphuris calcareum*. This also should be given in
various potencies, if several doses should be needed from time
to time. Often also, according to circumstances, a dose of ....
Mercury (in homœopathic preparation) may be used between."

So often homœopaths will baulk at the thought of giving
more than one remedy as part of the prescription, but as
Hahnemann developed his practice and gained by experience,
more and more he found the use of just one remedy too slow.
Though he may have given them to be taken at different times
or alternated, he would often use more than one remedy as
part of the same prescription. This is an issue which Rima

Handley discusses in her book, "A Homœopathic Love Story". On page 132 she mentions that Hahnemann "prescribed *Hepar sulph* orally every night to M. Uruchart, at the same time giving him a dose of *Merc sol* to inhale."

We live at a time when in England, a large proportion of our patients are walking around with teeth filled with amalgam which is approximately 50% mercury. Many of these patients display some symptoms included in the symptom picture of *Hepar sulph*, which leads us to prescribe it almost routinely after *Psorinum*, in descending potencies before the indicated remedy. Alternatively we sometimes use *Hepar sulph* at the beginning of the day, with a compatible indicated remedy given at the end of the day. This leads to a considerable improvement in many conditions where previously progress had been slow.

Results with Irritable Bowel Syndrome (IBS) led us to give a talk on our work to meetings of the IBS Network, which in turn led them to ask us to write an article for their newsletter. Part of the text of this is printed below:

"It is well known that IBS, along with many other western diseases is almost unknown in the third world. At least it was until western man moved in with his refined sugars, flours and processed foods.

Stress can be considered a trigger of IBS, but certainly not a cause, as the third world is far from being free of stress yet IBS is largely unknown. So does this put the blame solely on diet, or is there another factor? I became suspicious of the diet theory as I encountered more patients with IBS who had always been on a whole food diet and yet who had acquired the condition, or who had switched to a whole food diet with little or no improvement.

A little over two years ago I became aware of the missing factor when treating a dental nurse with IBS. Her symptoms had apparently begun shortly after taking up her post in which she mixed the mercury amalgam for tooth fillings. I studied the toxic effects of mercury and in particular some of the writings by J.G. Levenson, President of the British Dental Society for Clinical Nutrition. I was drawn to the following facts.

'When mercury vapour enters the saliva in people's mouths and is swallowed it will combine with hydrochloric acid to form mercuric chloride......Mercuric chloride will destroy gut bacteria and allow an overgrowth of candida and other yeasts. The formation of this compound may leave the body deficient in hydrochloric acid, thus digestion is not correctly initiated and cannot proceed efficiently.'

Symptoms of low level chronic exposure to mercury may vary enormously depending on the inherent resilience of the individual. Symptoms may occur at the time of placement of a filling or when an old amalgam is removed. More often, however, the effects are insidious, taking perhaps five years or more to show. This is an important feature as it goes part of the way in explaining why the release of mercury from fillings has not been generally accepted by the health professions as being implicated in disease. If a patient has fillings placed and five years later develops arthritis, migraine or is generally unwell, it is highly unlikely that a diagnostic correlation would be made by a physician.

An increasing volume of research evidence shows beyond dispute that:
1. Mercury is released from dental amalgam fillings.
2. It combines with tissues and continually accumulates.
3. It can affect the ability of the immune system to function.
4. It can have very severe effects on the health of human beings.
5. The presence of different metals in the same tooth or in different teeth act as a battery with the saliva as the electrolyte. The battery effect also releases mercury from the filling.

Obviously not everyone is sensitive to the effects of mercury and not everyone has the problem which we are now considering, but there is a wealth of material about gastro-intestinal trouble caused by mercury in industry.

So what happened in the third world? Western man brought his refined food causing tooth cavities and he also brought his dentists with their mercury and his doctors using mercurial preparations. The work "quack" is an abbreviation of 'quicksilver', another name for mercury, and quack doctors, as they were called, used mercury to suppress an inordinate number of symptoms.

Other reports show how mercury from the mother can travel through the blood stream and affect the unborn child. This means that even where the next generation has not received any fillings a degree of mercury poisoning may be present and give rise to IBS. There is also information to show that some people developed IBS and other symptoms after they had fillings removed and mercury leaked into the gut."

It is interesting to note how mercury from parents can affect their offspring. Research by Dr Murky J Viny, Professor of the University of Calgary in Canada has shown that when amalgam was placed in the teeth of sheep within a month, mercury was to be found in various tissues of the body including the liver and kidneys. Kidney function was reduced by 50% within 30 days of placement of the fillings. In pregnant sheep mercury crossed the placenta into foetal tissue and in nursing sheep their milk had eight times more mercury than did their blood.

This has resulted in us often using the remedy *Hepar sulph* with young children who have not received any mercury fillings, because there may well be an inherited dyscrasia or block to cure from the parent's fillings.

There are other remedies which are known for their ability to antidote the effects of mercury in the system. One is *Sulphur* which, as has been discussed, Hahnemann used to start many of his cases to deal with the inherited psoric miams, as well as working to antidote the effects of mercury in the system. However experience shows the inherited psoric miasm is modified by the sulphur and much of the power of the potentised medicine is used up by this, and there is little left to deal with the mercurial problem. This is probably one of the reasons why Hahnemann advocates the following of *Sulphur* by *Hepar sulph* in a prescription. This is illustrated in one of his cases when Mme Lelor was given *Sulphur* 30 followed by *Sulphur* 24, then *Hepar sulph* 24, then *Hepar sulph* 18 and then 12. ("Homœopathic Love Story" - Rima Handley).

We have illustrated much of our discussion about mercury with examples of digestive problems, but we would not wish to give a one sided picture. Mercury is one of the most toxic substances known to man. In the gut it can alter the chemical make up of the friendly bacteria so that it can no longer keep fungal infections such as candida albicans in check. In Alzheimer's disease there is evidence that mercury rather than aluminium is the highest trace element in the brain ("Brain Research", 553 1990 - research by W.R. Marksbery, University of Kentucky).

The effects of mercury poisoning can be identical to the symptoms of Alzheimer's disease (BBC Panorama 1994).

Evidence has shown that mercury is continuously released from fillings and the amount of vapour is increased when chewing especially hot or acidic foods. Symptoms may occur at the time of placement of a filling or when old amalgam is removed but often the effects are insidious. Some countries have banned the use of mercury. More recently Germany, Austria and Sweden are introducing moves to make mercury amalgam illegal.

Mercury can cause neurological, respiratory, cardiovascular and digestive disorders, be implicated in food, chemical and inhalant allergies and candida and other fungal proliferations. Common features include: chronic fatigue, feeling the cold excessively, tingling in limbs, tremor in hands, frequency of urination, irritability, depression, metallic taste in the mouth and increased salivation. Mercury can reduce the total and alter the ratio of T blood cells. T cells are crucial to the competence of our immune system.

Much of the population has amalgam fillings and whether they are outwardly affected or not depends of their own resilience or susceptibility to mercury. However everyone who has mercury fillings uses part of their immune system to cope with the mercury.

We have spoken much about mercury but there are other dyscrasias that can block the indicated homœopathic remedy from working as well as it might. A dyscrasia is a taint causing an artificial illness that the body's energy cannot throw off. This taint can come from a variety of origins; allopathic drugs for example can "poison" the body, and their effects can be felt for years afterwards. Sometimes the patient can tell you they have never felt well since such and such happened to them but often the dyscrasia is much more insiduous and can only be discovered by close questioning and deduction.These dyscrasias can prevent the body attaining good health and prevent well selected homœopathic remedies from working as they should. Many practitioners have had patients who have not responded as well as expected. As homœopaths we tend to think we have not found the similimum and go back to our materia medicas and repertories and find another remedy to try, and then another. Such remedy hopping is detrimental to the patient and can muddle up the case by altering the original symptom picture, it can also make us despair of homœopathy and our ability. In fact the first remedy we tried is often the correct one but has not been able to work because a dyscrasia is causing the blockage.

We no longer have to cope with the leeches and venesections of Hahnemann's day, (about which he writes in paragraph 74 of the Organon) but the drugs and pollutants of our modern world bring with it their own problems which can only be overcome if our energy is assisted by the right potentised medicines and then our indicated remedies may work efficiently and without hinderance.

Immunisations can also be a relevant factor. Whatever the measure of protection from immunisation, many people are not happy with the idea of injecting two month old babies, whose immune systems are still developing, with antigens straight into the blood stream. Research is indicating that the limited protection of immunisation is being bought at a cost of not just immediate affects, but long term dangers such as MS, cancer and even AIDS.

Research is proving that immunisations are having a negative impact on the genetic structure and the immune system which leads to chronic degenerative diseases later in life. It appears to interfere with the balance of helper and suppresser T-lymphocytes and this affects the allergic responses. ("Vaccination and Immunisation: Dangers, Delusions and Alternatives", Leon Chaitow)

Multiple sclerosis has been attributed to the measles vaccine and AIDS to the smallpox vaccine. Surveys of cot deaths show two thirds of those affected had received DPT vaccine in the previous 21 days. Many chronic diseases such as hypertension, diabetes, gout and Parkinson's have shown deterioration after injections for the prevention of flu.

The effect we are most likely to see in our consulting room is that of the allergy related illnesses - the eczemas, asthma, hay fever, chronic catarrh, glue ears. All these have reached epidemic proportions. Thirty years ago asthma was unusual and now it seems common place for a child to carry an inhaler in their school bag.

A survey detailed in the British Medical Journal showed that 6% of 12,500 children born in one week in 1958 had atopic eczema and by 1970, 12 years later, a similar survey showed that the figure had doubled. What would that figure be now? While this may be partly attributed to industrial pollution, car exhaust fumes, pesticides and chemicals in our food, this figure has increased in proportion to the increase in immunisations and when we see many complaints starting soon after an immunisation we realise there must be a link.

Often we can help such conditions with our indicated remedies, but for these to work effectively and to gain a lasting cure we will need to go back to the original dyscrasia and remove that. Kent in his lecture on the remedy *Thuja* stated that, "*Thuja* is a pre-eminently strong medicine when you have a trace of animal poisoning such as snake bite, small-pox or other vaccination". A snake bite is very like a vaccination, injecting a toxin straight into the blood stream. A vaccination causes the body to produce catarrh or other sycotic manifestations in order for the body to attempt to throw off its toxic overload, hence the relationship between *Thuja* and Sycosis. *Thuja* can therefore be used when there is a strong history of vaccinations and indicated remedies are not working or when there has been an obvious deterioration in health since a vaccination. Many cases of children with catarrh and glue ears will not have a permanent cure until *Thuja* is used.

We have many cases of catarrh, sinus problems and glue ear which have been cured without even giving a specifically indicated remedy but just using *Hepar sulph*, and *Thuja* for the dyscrasia and nosodes related to the basic miasms. *Psorinum* followed by *Hepar sulph* then *Thuja* and then *Tuberculinum* in descending potencies immediately following each other have produced the results. At other times *Psorinum* may have been used in descending potency followed by *Hepar sulph* 30 for five days at the beginning of the day, *Berberis* 30 in the afternoon to assist the elimation of toxins (as a drainage remedy) and *Thuja* 30 at the end of the day.

We do not give *Thuja* with quite the routineness of *Hepar sulph* because, although most people have been vaccinated in the past, there is not the ongoing exacerbating cause as with the continual slight leakage of mercury from the teeth. We may therefore give *Thuja* if sycotic symptoms are manifesting themselves, but it is not a remedy which we will usually need to regularly repeat.

On the other hand we have often seen eczema or a similar complaint clear up under homœopathic treatment, only to return with a vengeance after a MMR vaccination. *Thuja* and also sometimes the vaccination itself in the 30th potency have been needed before the case has had a totally satisfactory outcome.

We can sometimes obtain very pleasant surprises from dyscrasia treatment and see improvements in a patient that are not obviously covered by the symptom picture of the dyscrasia remedy being used. This may be because too little is known about the symptom picture of our dyscrasia remedies, or it may be that as the potentised medicines clear away a blockage to health the patients' vitality is able to increase so that it can eradicate a problem as best it knows how.

A case in point was Mrs J. She had a history of sepsis since an operation when a swab had been left in her abdomen. Various remedies showed some progress. However after *Psorinum* followed by *Pyrogen* in descending potencies not only did she make a considerable improvement, but her long lost sexual libido returned. *Pyrogen* is not a remedy known for this influence, it therefore appears to have removed a barrier to cure so that the patients own recuperative ability was able to do the rest.

Pyrogen dispels the belief that homœopathic remedies are made from plants and harmless substances. *Pyrogen* is a product of the decomposition of chopped lean beef in water which is allowed to remain in the sun for two or three weeks. Sanderson defined it as, "a chemical non-living substance formed by living bacteria, but also by living pus-corpuscles, of the living blood or tissue protoplasms from which these corpuscles spring". It is therefore highly septic in its crude state. In potency of 6c and above however, any toxic element has been removed leaving us with a substance which according to the Law of Similars is capable of curing a toxic or septic condition. In his lectures on *Pyrogen*, Kent states that it, "cures many complaints that date back to septic conditions" and he used it to treat puerperal fever and also to treat nephritis which could be traced back to a septic origin. *Pyrogen* is not well known as a kidney remedy, but here is an example of

Kent using it in a dyscrasia type way and not just because of its symptom picture.

A modern day dyscrasia, unknown to our classical fathers of homœopathy is that of hormones. Over the past thirty years or so women in particular have been bombarded with hormones. The contraceptive pill which overrides the reproductive hormones has been used at one time or another by the majority of women. We have many patients who have either not felt right since going on the pill or have never been right since coming off. Pre-menstrual tension symptoms will often start after coming off the pill. Figures show that the suicide rate is higher among pill users. It can cause depression, weight gain, migraines, vaginal infections and can contribute to diabetes and liver problems.

The use of hormone replacement therapy (HRT) is increasing daily and although many women are wary of it, for many in the medical profession it is the wonder drug of the nineties. It boosts oestrogen levels un-naturally to prevent menopausal symptoms. Originally the oestrogen was used on its own, but it was found that this increased the risk of endometrial cancer. In the U.S.A. women must legally be informed of the risks of cancer associated with HRT. Progesterone was then added to help prevent the cancer but the side effect of this can be bloating, weight gain, breast swelling and tenderness and depressive moods - symptoms which many women hope to alleviate on HRT. Studies have shown that prolonged use of HRT increases the risk of womb and breast cancer and may affect the absorption of vitamins.

The biggest selling points of hormone replacement therapy are prevention of heart disease and osteoporosis. Much of the evidence and research for this is controversial and as regards osteoporosis it has been found that once coming off HRT there is a rebound effect with rapid bone loss. ("Ongoing research of women in Massachusetts", New England Journal of Medicine, October 1993)

There is also the 'morning after pill'. This is a man-made oestrogen known as DES. Originally this was used to prevent miscarriages in the 1940's, daughters of women who used it then have been shown to have a higher incidence of vaginal cancer and cervical abnormalities - an inherited hormonal dyscrasia. ("Folliculinum - Mist or Miasm", Melissa Assilem)

Hormones are also invisibly present in our food. Not only are animals given hormones to increase their size but pesticides also contain certain hormones which are sprayed on the grains and vegetables that both we and the animals eat. These excess hormones are excreted through the kidneys into the urine and hence through the miracles of recycling back into our water supply; hormones cannot be easily filtered out and so we get another dose in drinking water. All these additional hormones deeply affect the health and fertility of the body and use up yet more of our immune system and healing ability as we try to cope with them.

The homeopathic remedy *Folliculinum* can be used to assist the removal of a hormonal dyscrasia. It is a fairly modern remedy made from oestone, a synthetic form of oestrogen. There have been no organised provings in potency but women have been proving it in its crude form for years.

If a patient has a history of hormone use and is now presenting with any hormone related symptom, or has never been well since hormone treatment or hormonal therapy has upset them at any time, there will probably be a dyscrasia sitting there which needs *Folliculinum* to move the case on. Of course the pill has been in existence for over 30 years now, and so there can be an inherited dyscrasia from patients whose mothers were on the pill before they were born.

Modern literature shows *Folliculinum* on its own having been effective in treating fibroids, post natal depression, congestive mastitis, thrush, endometriosis, ovarian cysts, pre-menstrual bloating and breast swellings and pre-menstrual migraines. ("Materia Medica of New Remedies", Julian)

Homœopaths very frequently treat pre-menstrual tension, particularly in women who have had problems related to the contraceptive pill, and we will therefore cite two fairly common cases.

The first was a lady born in May 1950 who, in common with her sister suffered from tiredness, suicidal depression, low self esteem and headaches before periods. She wanted to be alone and shut the door to the world at this time. She regularly burst into tears without knowing why. She had received many mercury teeth fillings during her life without any obvious bad effects but she also had migraines which had started about the same time as taking the contraceptive pill.

She was first given *Psorinum* in descending potency of 10M, 1M, 200, 30, 12 and 6 on a daily basis to deal with the psoric predisposition, followed immediately by *Hepar sulph* from CM down to 3c for the possible mercurial dyscrasia and also to help with the oversensitive nervous system. The provings of *Hepar sulph* show it to be one of our greatest remedies for extreme sensitivity of the body to the environment as well as extreme sensitivity of the emotions.

Sepia was the next remedy to be used for the symptoms before her period. Two main remedies used for hormonal problems are *Sepia* and *Pulsatilla*, these will be discussed in more detail in the Materia Medica. Her emotional state in desiring to be alone at this time rather than having reassurance, company and support pointed firmly towards *Sepia*. It was therefore used daily in the descending potencies of 10M, 1M, 200, 30, 18, 12, 6 to be followed immediately by *Tuberculinum* in a similar way.

So having been given *Psorinum, Hepar Sulph, Sepia* and *Tuberculinum* in descending potencies (this included one dose of *Syphilinum* CM before completing the *Hepar sulph*), she was seen again five weeks later. The PMT had improved and the violent symptoms were only showing for a day rather than a week, the headaches were less in intensity and she was coping with stress better. *Folliculinum* was now given in descending potencies with the result that the headaches ceased totally, the PMT was on a much better level and her periods became shorter and better in consistency.

If she needs further treatment it would be expected that the *Sepia* would work more effectively, as the *Folliculinum* has cleared the ground for it to work to its maximum effectiveness. The reason that *Folliculinum* was not given earlier in the prescription was that although the pill appeared to have been responsible for the start of her migraines, the fact that she shared so many symptoms with her sister inferred a more misamatic inheritance causing the problem and so the need initially for *Psorinum* and *Tuberculinum*.

Another woman born in 1973 had a grandmother, mother and two sisters all suffering from PMT and bad periods. She said that not only just before the periods but for much of the month she suffered from nausea, anxiety, tiredness and irritability. She wanted to run away and have lots of space with freedom from all friends. She said that whilst she had been fine before going on the pill, since coming off it she had become a Jeckell and Hyde character. She was wanting to eat bread and 'stodge' before periods, and suffered from palpitations of the heart with the commencement of periods.

As her problems were for much of the month we needed to make a degree of improvement quickly. She was therefore given *Psorinum* in descending potencies concertinered over two days (10M, 1M, 200 on day one and 30, 12 and 6 on day two). For the next five days she was given *Hepar sulph* 30 in the mornings for the sensitivity and any mercurial dyscrasia. In the afternoon she was given *Berberis* 30 as an organ remedy and in the evenings *Sepia* 30. *Sepia* included all her main symptoms, as did *Pulsatilla*, but *Sepia* seemed to best fit her mental and emotional state.

This week's course was followed by a week's gap without any medicines. During this time her body was able to utilise the remedies which she was given during that first week. Our experience is that often people are aware of more improvement after they have finished a course of remedies. (The exception to this is when people are consistently taking heavy drugs which can stop the effective action of the remedies.)

After the week's break she was given a similar type of course using *Folliculinum* descending over the first two days followed by *Folliculinum* 30 in the mornings, *Berberis* 30 in the afternoons and *Sepia* 30 in the evenings again followed by a week's gap.

Seen one month after her first interview she declared that she was a lot better, calmer and less depressed with less PMT. Her period had been much improved and substantially less painful. She had eaten more normally before her period and there had been no palpitations during the menstrual cycle.

After a further break of a week she was given one more course maximising the use of all the remedies by giving them at daily intervals in descending potencies. She received *Psorinum*, *Hepar sulph*, *Sepia*, *Tuberculinum* (to deal further with the miasmatic background) and then the deeper acting remedies of *Lycopodium* and *Silica* to deal with the hereditary predisposition.

After this she stated that she was fine, had no problems that needed further treatment and she also said that she felt her energy improved and that she had thrown off a cold quicker than normal.

Her prescription was a fairly typical one for many women in her position which to recap was as follows:-

Day 1	*Psorinum* 10M, 1M, 200
Day 2	*Psorinum* 30, 12, 6
Days 3 - 7	*Hepar sulph* 30 - morning;
	Berberis 30 - afternoon;
	Sepia 30 evening
Days 8 - 13	Nil
Day 14	*Folliculinum* 10M, 1M, 200
Day 15	*Folliculinum* 30, 12, 6
Days 16- 20	*Folliculinum* 30 - morning
	Berberis 30 afternoon
	Sepia 30 evening

One month later a second interview and prescribed remedies in descending potencies, one potency taken each day as follows:-

Psorinum 10M down to 6

Hepar sulph CM down to 3 with one dose of *Syphilinum* CM

Sepia 10M down to 6

Tuberculinum CM down to 6

Lycopodium 10M down to 3

Silica 10M down to 3

When looking at such a lengthy course as that given above, practitioners working on their own without a dispenser could be forgiven for throwing up their hands in horror and saying that they could never cope with the dispensing side of the work. With this we have great sympathy, but we would point out that you will get quicker, you will need to spend very little time working out with a repertory, (Hahnemann we are told rarely used one) and you will have satisfied patients which will promote the cause of homœopathy.

Until recently homœopathic research has normally been involved with the proving of more and more remedies. An increasing number of homœopaths are now asking for research working towards making an efficient use of our well known and trusted remedies which have been in use for decades. This is very much the theme of this book.

However there are certain dyscrasias which were not

around in Hahnemann's times and we need our remedies to match them. One such remedy, *Folliculinum*, we have just discussed. Another remedy is *Radium bromide*.

In 1898 Marie and Pierre Curie discovered an element which greatly eclipsed every other in radiating power and they appropriately gave it the name of radium. This element gives out light, heat and gases without apparently losing weight and it was soon seized upon by the medical world. X-rays were already in use at this time but radium soon became the dominant material used.

M & Mdm Curie were interviewed for "Pall Mall Magazine" of 17th October 1903, when they said, "The doctors think that they can cure lupus and polyps and perhaps cancer with it but I know nothing about that .... but it will burn. I can testify to that. I put a tiny bit of a salt of radium in an india rubber capsule, fastened it on my arm and left it there for ten hours. When I took it off the skin was red and the place soon turned into a wound which took four months to heal". This can be considered a proving and we therefore know that it will be a remedy dealing with the dyscrasias left by X-rays and X-ray burns.

In 1904 Dr John Clark started experimenting on healthy humans with a homœopathic preparation of *Radium* and for the first time we had information about the administration of the remedy. Symptoms produced included weakness, lassitude and tiredness which are all common results of the effects of radiation. Many people who spend hour after hour in front of a VDU will respond much better to homœopathic treatment after *Radium bromide* has been given in potency.

A colleague discovered cases diagnosed as myalgic encephelitis (M.E.) or Post Viral Syndrome all improved considerably after prescribing *Radium bromide*. He was practising in Wales in an area where many sheep and crops had been destroyed as they contained levels of radiation considered too high to be allowed to enter the food chain after the leakage of radiation from the Russian atomic energy reactor at Chernobyl had affected vast areas of land. That radiation was a factor in the health of these patients can understandably be surmised from the results of using this remedy.

Another area in which *Radium bromide* is able to break through many dyscrasias requires a basic knowledge of chemistry and in particular the periodic table of elements. Radium is a heavy element with an atomic weight of 88 and can, therefore, displace those elements in the same group of a lower weight. These elements include Barium (56), Calcium (20) and Magnesium (12).

Mr B was born in 1961 and came to see us suffering from permanent indigestion. He had been sent by his doctor to the hospital to have a barium meal X-ray. A small hiatus hernia was diagnosed and he was told that his stomach produced too much acid. He constantly dosed himself on Milk of Magnesia. The effect of alkaline tablets is to immediately settle the stomach but as the stomach should be an acid environment the result of these patent medicines is to improve the symptoms for a short time. The body, determined to maintain the status quo, pours in more acid in order to compensate and the result is a greater and greater reliance on magnesium preparations.

Mr B came with a burning in his oesophagus which he believed could be triggered by stress and at least three reasons for prescribing *Radium bromide* - firstly, the X-ray, secondly, the Barium and thirdly, the Magnesium preparation.

Even before being given the normal psoric remedies he was given *Radium bromide* to help with the heavy dyscrasia and his full prescription was as follows;-

Day 1	*Radium bromide* 10M, 1M, 200
Day 2	*Radium bromide* 30, 12, 6
Days 3 - 7	*Radium bromide* 30 - morning
	Berberis 30 - afternoon
	Nux vomica 30 - evening
Days 8 - 13	Nil
Day 14	*Psorinum* 10M, 1M, 200
Day 15	*Psorinum* 30, 12, 6
Days 16 - 20	*Hepar sulph* 30 - morning
	Kali phos 30 - afternoon
	Nux vomica 30 - evening

The *Hepar sulph* was prescribed because of his mercury fillings and the *Nux vomica* is indicated both by the symptoms present and by the stress factors involved. Mr B telephoned after completing his prescription to say that he no longer had any problem, neither did need to take any ant-acids.

Some practitioners consider the calcium tablets and calcium

fortified foods which are given to babies, growing children and adults, create their own problems as the calcium is given in higher doses than the natural balance and therefore works like a drug in the system causing its own dyscrasia. This makes *Radium bromide* a useful remedy at any age as it can help remove this excess calcium.

We have examples where we have used this remedy to help people after radiotherapy in cancer. Also for radiologists and dentists where the X-ray precautions may be poor, *Radium bromide* as a remedy can be very useful.

Miss J was a patient who for some months had suffered from post viral syndrome and had been given lengthy courses of anti-biotics to try to clear up both her primary chest infection and then any remaining sequelae. In her case before the indicated remedy of *Rhus tox* she received *Psorinum* followed by *Hepar sulph* followed by *Penicillinum*. The remedies were all given in descending potencies at 48 hour intervals until the patient began to improve and then at intervals of 24 hours. Giving the potencies at greater intervals allowed each strength to work longer and hence deeper in the system before the next potency came along to modify the action of the previous dose. We would not normally give the doses continually at intervals of more than a day at the beginning of treatment as we could be concerned about the remedies initially working deeply and causing initial discomfort before improvement.

Penicillinum is derived from Penicillin but is used in potency in order that it is totally non-toxic and works by stimulating the body's vitality. It is particularly useful when the vitality has been lowered as a result of taking antibiotics indiscriminately, destroying both good and bad bacteria. As homœopathic remedies work in accordance with the Law of Similars; *Penicillinum* is close enough to the symptomatology and effect of most antibiotics to work even if we are not dealing with a dyscrasia left by a penicillin based drug. An exception to this rule is Septrin, which needs to be given in potency if required.

We do not automatically give *Penicillinum* in potency because a patient has had antibiotics in the past any more that we would automatically give *Thuja* because a person had been vaccinated. However, if an individual's problems can be related to the effects of antibiotics then we know that this can impede the action of other remedies. There is a relationship of fungus/penicillin to the anaerobic/fungal elements of Candida which is often a factor in post viral syndrome and therefore we can help the body to overcome the proliferation of the fungal element.

We have now briefly reviewed the most common dyscrasias or barriers to cure. Others we meet occasionally. One such person had been working in the Middle East and had often inhaled crude oil fumes from oil wells. *Petroleum* was given in potency which expedited the action of the following indicated remedy. The potentised preparation is made from a trituration and tincture of the rectified oil. Coal tar is a related substance and where suppression has been caused by the topical applications of coal tar products, *Petroleum* in potency can be tried.

A dyscrasia may sometimes be caused by a trauma. For instance many popular first aid books on the market will reveal that *Arnica* is the foremost remedy for bruises. It is a plant which grows on the hills and mountains of Europe and if any animal loses its footing it seems instinctively to nibble this plant, which reduces the swelling and bruising. Sometimes we have a patient with no such symptoms but on careful questioning we find that their condition started a few weeks after a fall. Again we would normally give *Arnica* before our indicated remedy and expect success.

Ignatia is another trauma remedy, helping this time to restore emotional equilibrium after a shock such as the death of a friend or relative. This can be a time when we feel extremely low and can be susceptible to a number of physical complaints. The remedy will not take away our grief, but it can act as a handrail helping us to cope better, and may be given possibly after *Psorinum* and before *Hepar sulph* as the indicated remedy. As the higher potencies work more deeply and effect the emotional levels, so in these cases we would normally use the remedies in order of descending potencies to ensure that our remedies worked successfully on all levels.

One of the reasons for lack of success with remedies which cover the symptom picture and therefore should work curatively, is that their strength is used up by a barrage of obstacles. In this Chapter we have endeavoured to show how many of these obstacles can be removed to give our remedies a clear pathway to success.

Occasionally we will still find cases with no obvious dyscrasia and yet there still seems to be something blocking the total or partial success of our remedies. It is under these circumstances that we will descend our potencies at greater intervals than 24 hourly to allow each strength to work at a greater depth. When the patient begins to respond we will then normally again resume a daily dosage.

We would conclude this chapter by quoting from para 41 of "The Organon":

"The association and mutual complication of dissimilar natural diseases in the same body occur much less frequently than those disease complications that are the result of inappropriate allopathic treatment through the prolonged use of unsuitable medicines.

From the continual repetition of unsuitable medicines, new and often very chronic disease conditions corresponding to the nature of these drugs associate themselves with the natural disease being treated. ..... Gradually they combine with the dissimilar chronic trouble, complicating it, so that a new dissimilar artificial disease of chronic nature is added to the old one. Thus the patient who was simply ill is now double so, so much more ill and difficult to cure that he sometimes becomes incurable, often even dies."

CHAPTER THREE

———◦<>◦———

THE LAW OF SIMILARS REVISITED

The conventional and traditional view of homœopathy is that the main pillar of this system of healing is the 'Law of Similars'. In other words a disease producing certain symptoms in an individual will be cured by the use of a remedy which in its clinical trials was capable of producing like symptoms in a healthy individual.

In para 18 of "The Organon", Hahnemann states that, "the sum of all the symptoms in each individual case (of disease) must be the sole indication, the sole guide to direct us to the choice of remedy". Most homœopaths consider the mental and emotional states to be prime symptoms to take into account. Next in importance are the "I" symptoms e.g. I am tired, I like sweets etc., then we consider the particular symptoms. These are the "my" symptoms e.g. my throat is sore, or my skin itches.

These symptoms are elicited by 'provings'. This word

comes from the German word 'prufing' which means test or trial, rather than our English word 'proof'. There are over 2,000 remedies in our homœopathic materia medica. More remedies are being proved all the time. Some of these are foodstuffs, others can be animal, vegetable or mineral and some are definitely bizarre in their origins.

Hahnemann had a thriving successful practice using about thirty remedies. When we were at college we asked tutors why this was and why we had to know so many. We were told that Hahnemann, "knew how to use these remedies".

If we take the attitude that every homœopathic remedy has a slightly different symptom picture, a different emphasis, a different nuance then we can understand why we need to know in detail such a large number of remedies. However the precept of 'strange rare and peculiar' symptoms which is studied today, and learned in detail by homœopathic students brought up on "The Organon", is never mentioned in "Chronic Diseases". Hahnemann had moved away from this in all but acute diseases and preferred instead, to speak of psoric pictures.

We now rarely use more than about 30 remedies ourselves in chronic conditions, the reason being that we are making our remedies work better. We do this by clearing the way with miasmatic and dyscrasia remedies and then, if necessary by following the indicated remedy through with drainage and deeper acting remedies.

In paragraph 171 of "The Organon", Hahnemann hints at the view expressed in "Chronic Diseases", that every successive homœopathic remedy should be chosen "in consonance"; that is in harmony with the symptoms of the patient "remaining after the expiry of the action of the previous remedy".

When we lecture from "Chronic Diseases" and illustrate our lecture from Hahanemann's own case-notes, showing his use of more than one remedy as part of the same prescription, even though they are administered on different days, or at different times of day, we are always asked the same question. How do we know which remedy is working? The answer is simple; we know from the symptom picture - from the provings - which remedy is working, because we know what it is capable of doing. Our role is to ensure that it does what is required of it by paving the way for it to act effectively, and if necessary ensuring that it will do its work by taking it into greater depth. Therefore, if the body's recuperative ability is capable of bringing about a cure, we know that we can obtain the results.

So how do we maximise the use of our remedies in order to achieve the desired results? If we consult any record of provings it will become apparent that different symptoms were produced by the different potencies. This means that to prescribe just one potency is not using our remedy to its maximum potential. Another factor is that many of even our commonest remedies have only been seriously proved in two or three potencies. Their maximum potential, therefore, is virtually unknown. This fact reputedly led Kent, near the end of his life, to say that his Repertory (the most detailed work of its kind until recently) was so inadequate as to be almost worthless. Our remedies can encompass much more than is apparent from their known symptom picture.

In his book, "Materia Medica Pura", Hahnemann hinted at another valuable truth. Which is that every remedy in the different potencies will encompass its opposite modalities. For example *Pulsatilla* is generally known as a thirstless remedy, but it is also to be found in the repertories under the heading "thirsty". Similarly *Silica* which is generally known as being a chilly remedy is also to be found under the headings "hot" or "heated". Remedies having a desire for certain foods in their symptom picture will also, probably in other potencies, have an aversion to those same articles of diet.

In her book "Portraits of Homœopathic Remedies Vol 2", Catherine Coulter states when writing of *Nux vomica*,"Just as quadratic equations have both positive and negative roots, so also does the constitutional remedy have a two fold aspect".

This means that we spend less time than many conventional homœopaths seeking out peculiar symptoms, and modalities of symptoms because we know that our remedies can cover a full range of symptomatology when we use them in a full range of potencies.

CHAPTER FOUR

DRAINAGE

Straightforward cases where one homœopathic treatment will complete the cure in a chronic situation are becoming less and less common. Patients are increasingly full of the toxic effects of drugs, pollution, the environment and the by-products of abnormal nervous system and hormonal activity. More and more the homœopath needs to consider prescribing supportive remedies to help the body's channels of elimination. When a house is built, early priority is given to the drainage system and so it should also be when devising a treatment programme for the modern-day patient.

Remedies that are becoming more and more useful as cleansers of the system, to enable the indicated remedies to work include *Taraxacum* (kidneys, liver, pancreas, gall bladder), *Chelidonium* (liver), *Echinacea* (blood and lymph). *Berberis* (kidneys, liver, spleen and bowel), *Hydrastis* (bowel and mucous membranes), *Sarsaparilla* (kidneys, skin and blood stream) and *Ceanothus* (spleen).

"People's health in the future will be determined more by what toxins they can get rid of rather than what they can take in nutritionally", (Robert Davidson, Lecture on Environmental Pollutants). Release of miasmatic or acute poisons requires an efficient drainage system. This view was pioneered by Dr. Compton Burnett, and has been latterly researched by the late Pritam Singh.

Every mouthful we eat nowadays contains unnatural chemicals. Either they have been added directly to the food in order to preserve, flavour or colour it, or they have been added to the ground in which the crops grow in order to get more life out of a vitamin and mineral depleted soil, or have been applied as pesticides. They may be fed to farm animals either directly, for a variety of reasons or through polluted feed, or they may find their way into the food chain as general environmental pollutants caused by our present scant regard for the way we treat this planet. The human body was not designed with the capacity to breakdown and eradicate these substances.

Food eaten and worked upon by the various digestive enzymes leaves the small intestine and travels through the blood stream to the cells via the liver. It is the liver which must work as the body's 'sentry' to prevent harmful substances from entering and affecting the rest of the body, and it is the liver which acts as a biological 'processing plant', to break down these substances into ones less toxic which may then be allowed back into the bloodstream to be excreted by the kidneys.

It is not surprising that in the late twentieth century, diseases of the liver and the kidneys are on the increase so we shall briefly look at two remedies which tone up these organs and thus aid the body in its process of elimination.

The first of these is *Taraxacum officinalis* (Dandelion). The leaves of this plant affect the liver, and especially the kidneys, helping them to excrete their filtered load. While the root also affects the kidneys, its main sphere of action is on the liver, gall bladder, bile ducts and pancreas. Used herbally the leaves are a powerful diuretic but one which does not deplete the body of potassium, like most chemical diuretics, as the leaves are themselves a rich source of potassium and thus ingestion of this remedy leads to a net gain in the mineral. Used in potency however, *Taraxacum* acts dynamically through the vital force as an organ remedy and does not exert a direct physiological action. *Taraxacum* tincture and potencies made from the whole plant, feed, tone and support both the liver and the kidneys.

Clarke's "Dictionary of Materia Medica", mentions that the remedy aids biliousness, debility, diabetes, gall stones, gastric headaches, jaundice and liver affections, rheumatism and skin conditions. While this is an impressive list, it is completely understandable if it is appreciated that a remedy which aids in the processes of cleansing the liver and helping the kidneys excrete impurities will also cleanse the blood stream. The body will not therefore be using the skin as a major eliminative organ producing spots, pimples, etc. People with skin problems who have a very spicy diet will particularly benefit from *Taraxacum* as it is the liver which must turn strong spices into more benign substances.

In the process of curing rheumatic and skin conditions, aggravations are initially common, as the body is undergoing something of a spring clean. Just as when we sweep a dirty room dust can be stirred up; but as the sweeping continues the room becomes cleaner. However by using intercurrent remedies like Taraxacum in the 30th potency or below, aggravations can be minimised by providing an effective vent for the system's toxic load.

A similar remedy is *Berberis vulgaris* (Barberry), which has an affinity for the liver, kidneys, gall bladder, spleen and bowel, helping the removal of toxic bacteria from the latter. The crude herb or tincture is best avoided during pregnancy, but this is not a problem encountered when using the remedy in potency. Clarke's "Dictionary" lists biliousness, bladder affections, dysmenorrhoea, fistulae, gallstones, urinary calculi and gravel, jaundice and liver problems, rheumatic and joint problems, tumours, leucorrhoea and lumbago amongst the conditions helped. Again the body forms stones around debris in the system, although there is often an inherited predisposition to calculus formation.

Berberis and *Taraxacum* may be used interchangeably or alternately, though we must take into account that *Taraxacum* is made from the whole plant including the root whilst *Berberis* is made from the tincture of the root bark. Homœopathy is not the law of identicals. A reading in a full materia medica may help the homœopath distinguish between these two remedies but whichever we use we are likely to produce a smoother path to recovery in cases characterised by toxicity than would otherwise be the case.

More and more, 'classical homœopaths' are having difficulty making their remedies effective in our polluted world and many are trying to devise different strategies in order to attempt to overcome this problem. One such person is Dr Ivo Bianchi, who recently wrote an article in the magazine "Biological Therapy" (vol. XI, 1993) entitled, "Allopathy, Homœopathy, Homotoxicology: An Outline". In this article he quotes Dr Hans-Heinrich Reckeweg who, writing in the 1930's, claimed that illness was not always caused by an inherited or constitutional condition but was often a result of the body reacting to, "the presence of toxins in the organism". He claimed that Hahnemann was thinking along very similar lines in "The Organon". Dr Bianchi added that, "Clearing the pathobiography of the patient is often essential for creating a rational therapeutic plan". In other words, homœopaths must have a strategy, and that strategy must include helping the body in its process of elimination, and he considered that such remedies which helped the body in this also helped the classic constitutional remedies to complete their action on a functional and pathological level. Toxins may be inhaled or ingested, may be the result of cell metabolism, and may often be by-products of deranged nervous and hormonal activity.

Moreover, De Bianchi criticises classical homœopathy because it relies too much on the practitioner's intuition and often comes to a diagnosis based on unreliable symptoms - as some of the symptoms are inherited and constitutional and others a result of pollution in the internal or external environment. He says, "It is almost impossible to heal serious and deep diseases only through stimulation of the vital force as provided by the administration of a single remedy with high dilutions given at long intervals".

The largest eliminative organ of the body is the skin. The dermal cells of all animals probably serve some excretory function, though this is most obvious with mammals. The sudiferous glands secrete large quantities of liquid which mainly consists of water, salts and urea. Perspiration appears to have the dual function of temperature regulation and excretion.

Elder is one of the most important herbal diaphoretics which, by increasing the elimination of toxins through the skin helps cleanse the body, and also reduce perspiration, and is an important but under-used remedy in homœopathy. The homœopathic potency, *Sambucus nigra*, is made from a tincture of the fresh leaves and flowers of the elder tree and, as would be expected, perspiration is one of the leading symptomatic indications for the prescribing of this remedy. Clarke's "Dictionary" states that, "We are often led to this remedy when we find a great deal of perspiration occurring with any other trouble, which may last all the time or it may come and go in paroxysms; it is sometimes found in phthisis; perspiration with disinclination to undress or be uncovered; heat with inclination to be covered".

Clinically, *Sambucus* is listed for angina, asthma, coryza, cough, croup, emaciation, catarrhal headaches, hoarseness, hydrocele, ileus, laryngismus, perspiration. pthisis, snuffles, whooping cough, etc. It is not a remedy to use for eczema and skin conditions as in these circumstances the skin needs to rest and remedies such as *Berberis* and *Taraxacum* should be considered to help channel toxins through the kidneys, etc. However, we have found many cases of asthma, catarrhal snuffles and suppressed breathing problems where the classically indicated remedies acted much more effectively after *Sambucus* had been given in potency. Suppressed skin conditions can lead to asthma. We would normally use *Berberis* as an initial drainage remedy. But after stimulating the kidneys as the main excretory organs, in order to help the body and blood stream filter its toxic load, we could then use *Sambucus* to encourage improved functioning of the skin with a resulting marked improvement in asthmatic conditions.

We normally use *Sambucus* either intercurrently in descending potencies, or in the 30th potency for 5 days periodically. Using descending potencies is in accordance with Hering's 'Law of Cure', as the vital force is being helped to work on the inherited and congenital, the mental and emotional levels and then to vent related impurities on the organ/functional level.

Where the skin is the main source of pathology, *Sarsaparilla* is to be used in preference. In material potencies it is a diaphoretic, alterative and anti-rheumatic. Many rheumatic conditions are caused by the body expelling its toxic load towards the extremities, and therefore a remedy assisting the kidneys and bloodstream is likely to help in rheumatic complaints.

Phatak states that *Sarsaparilla* in potency has its chief action on the genito-urinary organs and the skin. He says that it clears the complexion and is effective in rheumatism. It is one of the deeper acting homœopathic remedies, being made from the root and rhizomes, which are rich in mineral salts. Because of its depth of action, Phatak's "Materia Medica" states that it meets syphilitic, sycotic and psoric constitutions, it is also a remedy which can help the vital energy to overcome potential dyscrasias. It is a "restorative and blood purifier after exhausting courses of mercury". Although mercury is no longer used as a drug by the medical profession, the potential for the occurrence of severe mercury related problems still exists owing to its use in dental fillings as has been discussed. As a blood purifier *Sarsaparilla* will complement *Thuja* in aiding the body to overcome vaccinations and suppressed gonorrhoea dyscrasias.

Unlike *Berberis* and *Taraxacum*, *Sarsaparilla* is not a remedy which will necessarily assist the liver. We usually use it at a later stage in the treatment, when a more profound drainage remedy is needed.

The function of that strange organ the spleen is the production of lymphocytes, which manufacture antibodies, to filter out the worn out and infirm erythrocytes and to destroy bacteria or parasitic organisms that pass through it. Compton Burnett was one of the first homœopaths to realise the importance of *Ceanothus* as an organ remedy. Its usefulness is increasing and below is reproduced part of an article from, "New, Old and Forgotten Remedies", first published in 1906.

"This remedy has in practice, amply justified Dr. Burnett's recommendation in diseases of the spleen in 1887. It belongs to the natural order Rhamnaceae of the buckthorns. It is indigenous to the Northern States, and is there known as New Jersey Tea, Red Root and Wild Snowball. The tincture is prepared by maceration from the fresh leaves pounded into a pulp."

In the third edition of his, "New Remedies", Dr E.M. Hale first introduced *Ceonothus*, citing testimony from old school and Eclectic sources as to its value in inflammations and enlargement of the spleen, and adding to the statement which suggested to Burnett its homœopathicity to these morbid conditions, namely that: "In chronic cases when the spleen is no longer tender, under the use of *Ceanothus* tincture it soon becomes painful and tender and then shrinks rapidly to its normal size."

Dr Burnett's contributions to the pathogenetic effects on those to whom it had been given are:

1. *Ceanothus* frequently relaxes the bowels, even to the extent of diarrhoea.

2. An intelligent young lady, aged 26, had been taking *Ceanothus*, four drops thrice daily, with great benefit, when: "One day I felt great nervous excitement, with chilliness, loss of appetite, and such a shaky condition of the nerves that I could scarcely hold a knife and fork at dinner. I shivered with cold chills down the back". She discontinued the medicine, and all these symptoms ceased. Resuming the *Ceanothus*, they reappeared. Some diarrhoea ensued. The menses subsequently came on profusely, ten days too early, an unprecedented event in her experience.

3. Dr Fadnestock of the United States, proved *Ceanothus* upon himself, and found that it caused a sticking pain in the spleen followed by enlargement of that organ, worse on motion and rendering him unable to lie upon his left side. Following these symptoms came similar symptoms in the liver. The urine was greenish, frothy, alkaline; specific gravity 1030, and showed the presence of bile, with traces of sugar.

Ceanothus not only relieves deep-seated pain in the region of the spleen, without affecting any other part of the body as a rule, but it actually reduces a chronically enlarged spleen and seems to renovate a constitution which has broken down and has contracted pseudo heart disease, chronic cough, leucorrhoea, dyspepsia and attacks of dyspnoea. I now condense the reports of a few typical cases of cure:-

Case 1 (Burnett) - Lady suffering from acute splenitis. The symptoms were violent vomiting, cough with expectoration, pain all up the left side, profuse sweats and fever. For three weeks the patient was treated as for pleura-pneumonia, the spleen not having been percussed by the orthodox doctors, but without effect. After a careful examination, the spleen being found to be large and tender *Ceanothus* 1x cured in ten days.

Case 2 (Burnett) - A servant aged 55 suffering from palpitations and violent attacks of dyspnoea was found to have both spleen and liver greatly enlarged. She had been ill from ague thirty years before this. Splenic dullness extended to the left mamma and she could not bear even the pressure of her clothes. Five weeks of *Ceanothus* 1x relieved all her symptoms, even the left side pain which had lasted 25 years. Drinking anything cold brought on the dyspnoea. *Ceanothus* 1x for two months more completed the cure.

Case 3 (Anon from the Clinique, January 1901) - Mr V. aged 31, came August 23, 1900, stating that he had contracted malarial fever eight months previously. Quinine controlled the ague, but continual pain in the left side and back remained. He was tired and exhausted all the time losing flesh, perspiring easily, has a cough which increases the left side pain, this pain being worse in wet and cold weather. Without distinct periodic rigors, there is still frequently a chilliness down the back, and slight fever-ishness at irregular intervals.

The spleen was found much enlarged, and tender to press. Ceanothus, three drops every three hours, improved him greatly in a week; in three weeks all enlargement and tender-ness of the spleen had disappeared and the patient was well.....

We certainly owe to Burnett the knowledge of how to apply *Ceanothus* in diseases of the spleen, and even in deep-seated pain in the left hypochondrium not dependent on splenic enlargement.

Hydrastis canadensis is also known as golden seal or orange root; the remedy being made from a thick knotty yellow peren-nial underground stem. The plant was used a a tonic and restorative by theNative Americans, but it is now nearly extinct in the wild though it has been widely cultivated.

Its excretory function is mainly through the gut and it assists the body to remove from the bowels toxic bacteria.

Excretion through the gut lining or glands associated with the gut is a vital form of elimination and *Hydrastis* will aid this. It helps with regulating peristaltic activity and improving muscle tone as well as normalising gastric secretions. Because of this it has a reputation for helping both constipation and diarrhoea and is often used in low potency to help the constipation of the elderly.

Where gastric detoxification is needed, *Hydrastis* is an excellent remedy. It has a reputation for being tonic, antiseptic, restorative and soothing. It favourably influences digestive processes improving the appetite where necessary. As well as helping with acute gastritis it is one of the best remedies for long standing stomach problems especially where there is weakness and emaciation. It also has a reputation in helping with catarrh as it helps the body to eliminate toxins through more acceptable channels. Being a root it is a deeper drainage remedy than some of the other plant remedies and therefore rarely a remedy with which to start.

One last remedy which completes our list of drainage medicines is *Echinacea* or purple cone flower. This remedy is made from the tincture of the whole fresh plant and affects the glands and bloodstream. It detoxifies the blood and can be used where sepsis and toxic blood is a key factor. It is used frequently by herbalists and can be used to tidy up and especially to deal with the toxic effects caused by antibiotics - antibiotic by definition means anti-bacterial. *Echinacea* can be termed as a probiotic in that it assists the good bacteria in their scavenging work. It also has proven anti-viral properties. In this way *Echinacea* is very useful where the immune system is depleted, such as in cases of post viral syndrome. Here it will prevent the body succumbing to numerous viral infections where the resistance is low. It does this by helping the blood stream and glandular system to excrete its toxic load. Blood poisoning, septicaemia, bites and boils and microbial infections are all helped by this remedy.

When looking for deeper acting drainage mineral analogues, Pritam Singh chose two remedies; *Kali Phos* and *Causticum*. From his own biological and chemical research he concluded that the potassium and phosphoric elements of *Kali phos* were necessary for kidney and liver functions and it could be described as a deeper version of *Berberis*. It also acts deeply on the lymphatic and glandular system. *Causticum* has much in common with *Kali phos* in its chemical make up but again the addition of heat deepens its action and many stubborn toxic cases have improved after *Causticum* has been administered.

Osteo-arthritis case:

Women born January 1945. Heart problems, depression and cancer in the family background. Arthritis on father's side.

30.9.93 - Pain began in the spine 4 years ago following bruise and got worse recently. Fatigue. Lethargy. Stiffness of all joints. Worse from damp and cold. Much catarrh. Ache in back of neck and slight headache. Skin rashes. Was a trained dancer.

Remedies given in descending potency daily:-*Psorinum, Hepar Sulph, Berberis, Rhus Tox, Tuberculinum.*

The catarrh which is one sign of a build up of toxins in the system was one reason for using *Berberis* in descending potencies.

30.10.93 - 50% improved. Less fatigue. No headaches. Not so hungry. More well being. Kidneys more efficient. Stiffness a lot better. Some hand joint pains - this proved to be a return of old symptoms and thus considered to be a good sign. Skin eruption had gradually lessened. Back of neck much improved. Cold weather not so uncomfortable.

Remedies again given in descending potencies:- *Lycopodium, Silica* and *Carbo animalis*.

12.12.93 - Better in self. Emotionally clearer in mind. Not now having bouts of depression. A few spots, nodules came and went. Increase in bowel and bladder function. Return of old liver symptoms relating to past hepatitis. Great improvement in lower part of spine. Joint pains gone.

Remedies were then given for one week as follows:-

Day 1	*Radium bromide* 10M, 1M and 200 at hourly intervals.
Day 2	Nil
Day 3	*Radium bromide* 30, 12, 6 at hourly intervals

Days 4 - 8   *Radium bromide* 30 at 8am, *Symphytum* 30 at 2pm and *Ledum* 30 at 8pm. *Ledum* was used because of bone changes.

11.1.94 - Joint pains and spine good. No pains. Skin good now. Liver fine. Bowels and urine fine. Much better generally.
Remedies given as follows:-

Day 1   *Psorinum* 10M, 1M and 200 at hourly intervals.
Day 2   Nil
Day 3   *Psorinum* 30, 12 and 6 at hourly intervals.
Days 4 - 8   *Hepar sulph* 30 at 8am, *Taraxacum* 30 at 2pm and *Symphytum* 30 at 8pm.

Taraxacum was used as it is deeper acting than *Berberis* with a particular affinity to the liver and kidneys.

24.2.94 - "Wonderfully well". Working longer hours. Sleeping well. No pain. Looser joints. Energy much better. Not depressed. Skin fine. Temporary return of foot rash.

Eczema Case

Boy born March 1990. Tuberculosis, asthma, eczema and psoriasis in the family.

29.3.94 - Had eczema for 3 months. Dry eczema aggravated by hot baths. Changeable moods. Very sensitive. General health good. History of multi-vitamins and minerals.
Remedies:

Radium bromide descending from 10M over two days.

Days 3 - 7   *Calc carb* 30, *Berberis* 30 and *Rhus tox* 30
Days 8 - 14   Nil
Days 15 and 16   *Psorinum* descending from 10M over two days.
Days 17 - 21   *Rad brom* 30, *Kali phos* 30 and *Pulsatilla* 30

Kali phos is deeper acting that *Berberis* which will also assist with stress related symptoms.

29.4.94 - Has had chickenpox but exceptionally mildly compared to other members of the family. Eczema has gone as has the itching leaving just a little dry skin. Much better before second course started. No need of any more treatment at present. No remedy given for now but remedies given to hold in case of return of symptoms:-

Psorinum 10M descending over two days.

75

| Days 3 - 7 | *Hepar sulph* 30, *Kali phos* 30 and *Rhus tox* 30. Would consider *Tuberculinum* if further treatment is needed. |

Chemically Related Eczema Case
Man born June l971

20.5.94 - Dry skin on hands could be chemically related. Spots vesicles under the skin which weep and discharge. Itches and stiff. Water aggravates. Started four years ago. Started on one finger. Last 3 months worse. Chemicals aggravate. Stress does not affect it. Wind aggravates. Perspires a lot. Warmth aggravates.

Remedies:

Psorinum descending from 10M over two days.

Day 3 - 7	*Radium bromide* 30, *Berberis* 30 and *Rhus tox* 30
Days 8 - 14	Nil
Days 15 and 16	*Sulphur* 10M descending over two days.
Days 17 - 21	*Hepar sulph* 30, *Kali phos* 30 and *Rhus Tox* 30.

23.6.94 - Started to improve during the first week then worsen. Now less weepy and less large spots. More itchy in last few days and stiff with heat.

Remedies:

Radium bromide descending from 10M over 2 days

| Days 3-7 | *Thuja* 30, *Echinacea* 30, *Rhus tox* 30 each day. |

Echinacea was used to assist with the blood stream and cleansing the lymph system.

Days 8 - 21	Nil
Days 22 - 23	*Tuberculinum* 10M descending in two days.
Days 24 - 28	*Radium bromide* 30, *Kali phos* 30, *Lycopodium* 30.

20-7-94 - Cancelled as hands perfect.

Case - Glue Ear and Ear Infections
Boy born 30.11.91. Parents both had a history of ear problems. Mother has fish allergy. Sister Down's Syndrome. Hypothyroid and allergic rhinitis in family.

29.6.94 - Heart murmur. Glue ear. Ear Infections every time he is teething. Today he has a temperature (102) and was screaming in pain the previous night. Hearing appears normal. Colds always go to ears. He is off his food and drink when his ears are bad. Left ear is red.

As an acute prescription he was given *Psorinum* 10M descending followed by *Pulsatilla* 10M descending, followed by *Calc carb* 30, *Berberis* 30 and *Pulsatilla* 30 for five days.

Week two   Nil.

Week 3
Days 1 - 2   *Radium bromide* descending from 10M.
Days 3 - 7   *Radium bromide* 30, *Kali phos* 30, *Thuja* 30

20.7.94 - Fine after the first week so no remedies were given for three weeks.

Week 4
Days 1 - 2   *Tuberculinum* 10M descending over two days.
Days 3 - 7   *Hepar sulph* 30, *Thuja* 30, *Kali phos* 30.

8.9.94 - Fine; did not need to be seen again.

CHAPTER FIVE

———◦<>◦———

SOUNDING THE DEPTHS

Scattered about the classical homœopathic literature are refer-
ences to the depth of action of remedies. This information is
little used by British homœopaths, but does it have a place?
Experience shows that often we take a case so far and then
progress stops. We re-examine the symptom picture and try to
find a new more accurate remedy. However, as no remedy
seems clearer we may start to use our apparently second best
remedy or possibly another nosode. Soon we find little
improvement in the symptomatology and the patient becomes
more distressed and disillusioned, with the practitioner hopping
from one remedy to another and losing sight of the horizon.

When conditions are cured by the use of the indicated acute
or constitutional remedies, this means that those remedies have
been able to enter sufficiently deeply into the life force or
metabolism of the individual to deal with the disharmony in
their internal environment and no further action is required.

However, not infrequently when dealing with the patient's

condition, we are also dealing with their inheritance. For instance a baby might have just developed eczema but we know that the father had eczema or asthma, the grandfather many allergies and the great grandfather tuberculosis. There will come a point when our indicated remedies cease to be effective until we have given deeper acting remedies to match the depth of the disease.

When chronic conditions appear at mid-life these may be caused entirely by lifestyle or they may be inherited from the parents and similarly when conditions arrive in later life it is commonly found that these have been inherited from grandparents or from further back in the ancestry. We need to match this depth by the miasmatic action and depth of our remedies.

Let us consider a patient who comes to us with a digestive disorder. If the complaint is brought on by everyday stress, *Nux vomica* is a remedy to consider. Phatak states in his "Materia Medica":

"*Nux Vomica* is an everyday remedy. It corresponds to many diseased conditions to which modern man is prone to. It is useful to those persons who lead a sedentary life doing much mental work: or to those who remain under stress and strain of prolonged office work, business cares and worries. Such persons in order to forget their worries are apt to indulge in wine, women, rich stimulant food and sedative drugs; and ill effects from which they are apt to suffer. The typical *Nux* patient is rather thin, spare, quick, active, nervous and irritable. It affects the nerves causing hyper-sensitiveness and over impressionability - mentally and physically. Produces digestive disturbance, partial congestion and hypochondriacal states".

We can readily see that whilst *Nux vomica* will be likely to help and often cure the heartburn and indigestion brought about by business cares and worries, it is not a deep acting remedy.

If the patient has stomach ulcers which are inherited from parents and grandparents, *Nux vomica* may be the place to start to deal with the environmental and nervous factors but very soon we would need to move on to deeper remedies like *Lycopodium*, an intercurrent remedy, and then to *Podophyllum* which has often helped to deal with grosser pathology than *Nux vomica*.

In the diagram below we see the patient's symptoms portrayed by the first triangle. Three courses of treatment were given using miasmatic, dyscrasia, drainage remedies and remedies indicated on the symptom picture. All the prescriptions improved and eventually cleared up the condition without the need to tackle any inherited predisposition.

Fig 1

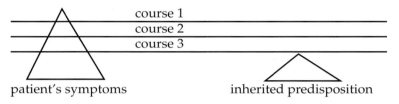

patient's symptoms   inherited predisposition

The following diagram, Fig 2, shows an improvement on the first two courses but the third course showed very little initial improvement and then a slight exacerbation of the problem. It was not that the condition had deteriorated but rather that the latent inherited predisposition had been uncovered and deeper acting remedies were necessary to work at a more profound level. By deeper we do not mean that there is anything harsh or drastic about the workings of these remedies. but rather that they will work gently and insidiously and often more slowly under the surface to bring about improvement in stubborn conditions.

Fig 2

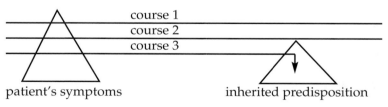

patient's symptoms   inherited predisposition

The last diagram, Fig 3, portrays a situation whereby the condition arose entirely from the inherited tendency. This may be the case of a baby born with eczema, which was a problem that the parents also suffered. On the other hand it may be someone who inherited rheumatism later in life. Her parents suffered from the condition but with her it remained latent until triggered by another condition, stress, poor nutrition, etc.

Fig 3

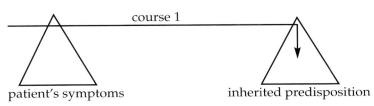

course 1

patient's symptoms   inherited predisposition

Here the first course has been extended using those deeper remedies before noticing any substantial improvement.

Pritam Singh observed that so often if a person showed symptoms in the first third of life, these were conditions caused by environmental and nutritional factors. Conditions arising after the age of 30-35 were often inherited from parents, whilst problems arising after the age of 60-65 were often to be found in the grandparents or even further back.

It has, therefore, been possible to roughly tabulate our commonly used remedies according to their depth of action. Generalisations are by definition full of inaccuracies but we have found it to be a useful working model.

Symptoms of Present Life
Level 1: *Aconite, Arnica, Baptisia, Belladonna, Coffea, Gelsemium, Ignatia*
Level 2: *Ledum, Nux vomica, Pulsatilla, Rhus tox, Sepia*

Symptoms of Parents (Age 30-35+)
Level 3: *Cocculus, Lycopodium, Phytolacca, Thuja*
Level 4: *Conium, Guaiacum, Nitric acid*

Symptoms of Grandparents (Age 60-65+)
Level 5: *Carbo veg, Graphites, Natrum mur, Natrum sulph, Podophyllum, Skookum Chuck, Wiersbaden*
Level 6 : *Alumina, Arsenicum album, Arsenicum sulphur flavum, Carbo animalis, Causticum, Fluoric acid, Radium bromide, Silica, X-Ray*

We see our first rung remedies as the short, sharp, acute acting remedies such as *Ignatia* for acute grief and other emotions; *Aconite* for acute fear or the beginnings of an acute cold; *Arnica* for an acute physical trauma; *Belladonna* for an acute fever; and *Baptisa* with an acute more septic fever with prostration.

Many of us have failed to cure a case because we have given a deep seated constitutional remedy for a very acute condition. Alternatively many a chronic case has not been cured because we have given too acute and superficial a remedy. Remedies can be given for their depth of action as much as for their symptom picture and to pitch at the right level will earn much gratitude from a patient.

There are numerous books on the market which show a relationship of remedies and also refer to their duration of action. Whilst there are question marks over the accuracy of such a generalised table, it is interesting to note that the duration of *Aconite* is listed in hours; *Belladonna* 1 - 7 days; *Ignatia* 9 days; *Arnica* 6-10 days; *Coffea* 1-7 days; and *Baptisia* 6-8 days, ("The Clinical Relationship of Remedies", P. Sankaran). This contrasts with our deeper, slower acting plant remedies such as *Conium*, listed as 30-50 days; and our deeper mineral remedies such as *Silica*, listed as 40-60 days.

Gelsemium is shown on the second line of this diagram. It is not generally a deep acting constitutional remedy, nor is it one for the sudden conditions which arrive with the immediacy of *Aconite*. More it is a remedy for the influenza's or the nervous stomach upsets which gradually build up over a few days. Rather than the person with a virus who produces an immediate temperature of 102-3 degrees and immediately needs *Belladonna*, with *Gelsemium* there is a low grade lingering fever of 99-101 degrees, the pace is generally slower.

Then we see the more constitutional remedies of *Nux vomica, Pulsatilla, Rhus tox,* etc., and so we continue down the scale to those remedies which work deeper and deeper dealing with long standing, stubborn and inherited conditions.

The depth of action of a remedy is learned from the symptomatology and conditions with which it can deal, its duration of action in the system, our own experience and the experience of other classical writers such as James Tyler Kent. One observation which we can make as we study this is that our more acute or superficial remedies are made generally from the aerial parts of plants, (e.g. *Nux vomica* from a nut, *Rhus tox* from leaves, *Ignatia* from seeds). Other, deeper, remedies are generally made from the whole plant or the roots which are obviously closer to the mineral salts in the soil. For instance of the root remedy *Podophyllum*, Kent writes, "This remedy is seldom used except in acute affections, but it is a long acting and deep acting drug; it produces a powerful impression on the economy; it relates to the deep-seated miasms."

Rhus tox comes from the leaves of a plant with comparatively shallow roots. *Guaiacum* has much in common with the symptomatology of *Rhus tox*. They both share similar rheumatic pains and chest problems. The remedy *Guaiacum* is made from the gum resin of a large tree with relatively deep roots and, as may be expected, is a deeper acting remedy which follows *Rhus tox* well and extends its action; it also antidotes any over-reaction from *Rhus tox*. Kent says of it, "This is a very deep acting remedy, even deep enough to cure the symptoms of and turn into order a constitution that is rheumatic, gouty and has inherited phthisis." He later goes on to say, "In psoric cases, complicated with syphilis and mercury and other violent drugs we find use for this most neglected remedy." Our bodies try to protect the vital organs such as the heart and lungs by throwing toxic waste towards the extremities and this is one factor conclusive to a rheumatic state. With mercury in so many people's systems as a result of slight leakage from amalgam teeth fillings, *Guaiacum* is another valuable remedy dealing with a constitution deeply affected by mercury poisoning.

We cannot consider the depth of action of remedies without also taking into account their pace of action. For instance, Socrates is reputed to have gradually poisoned himself with hemlock (Conium maculatum). The provers of *Conium* developed symptoms not immediately but very gradually. Hence the remedies where the symptoms developed slowly can be used to treat those conditions which have developed slowly and insidiously under the surface. Kent says of *Conium*, where the remedy is taken from the whole plant, including the roots, "This medicine is a deep, long acting antipsoric, establishing a state of disorder in the economy that is so far reaching and so long lasting that it disturbs almost all the tissues of the body."

But he goes on to talk of, "gradually growing" symptoms, "a general slowing down of all the activities of the body" and, "such a deep action that it gradually brings about certain states of mind".

When we go to the mineral based remedies, we have prescriptions with deeper action still and which are capable of stimulating the body to deal with deeper pathology. A look at the remedies which Samuel Hahnemann included in the materia medica part of his work, "Chronic Diseases", shows that a very high proportion of the remedies he mentions are derived from minerals. This is in keeping with the tone of his work as chronic diseases tend to be deep seated conditions for which there was often an inherited tendency.

For instance of Silica, Kent says, "Such are the long-acting, deep-acting remedies, they are capable of going so thoroughly into the vital order that hereditary disturbances are routed out". A few paragraphs later he writes, "It is the natural complement and chronic of *Pulsatilla*, because of its great similarity, it is a deeper more profound remedy." *Pulsatilla* is, of course, a plant remedy whereas *Silica* is a mineral.

We rarely would commence a prescription using a deep acting mineral remedy as the indicated medicine. We could find very little response as the case needs to be prepared to receive our deeper medicines. Alternatively we could find too much response. the body could be stimulated to throw out too much toxic material too soon to the discomfort of the patient. If a feather duster is needed we shouldn't begin with a scrubbing brush. Again Kent stated, "There are cases that would be greatly injured by so deeply acting a remedy as *Silica* if given in the beginning, that is the suffering would be unnecessary; but if you commence with *Pulsatilla* you can mitigate the case and prepare it to receive *Silica* ......"

A remedy which complements and follows *Silica* well is *Fluoric acid* and a study of *Fluoric acid* in the materia medica furnished us with information of gross and destructive pathology, necrosis and severe problems of bone, skin and brain. This is very different from the functional symptomolgy of *Pulsatilla*. Severe pathological changes take time to develop and we are therefore going to need to match this with remedies which are slow and deep acting. As we again quote Kent, this time on

Fluoric acid, note his comments regarding pace of action:

"It takes a long time for this remedy in the proving to develop its symptoms. It is a very deep-acting medicine and an antipsoric, anti-syphilitic and anti-sycotic. It is insidious in its action and its symptoms are slow in approach; it is like the deepest and slowest and most tedious diseases, the miasms, and hence it is suitable in the very slowest and lowest forms of disease."

It is true that deep acting remedies like *Podophyllum* and much more so, *Silica*, can be effectively used in acute disease (e.g. diarrhoea and abscesses respectively), but here the remedy is used up by the body's energy in dealing with the acute problem leaving little or none of the remedy left to continue to work with the miasmatic depths.

When dealing with distressing situations or conditions where the roots of the disease are in the family background, we need to commence with the indicated plant remedy, or sometimes, with a remedy with an animal poison such as *Sepia* made from the inky juice of the cuttle fish, or *Lachesis* made from a snake venom and then progress, often through a remedy made from a root or whole plant, to a related mineral remedy which fits the symptom picture and has a good follow on or complementary relationship. Where no remedy is obvious we may use one such as *Wiersbaden* or *Skookum Chuck*. These are both prepared from mineral-rich water containing many deep acting ingredients in solution and in balanced combination.

Natrum mur is a widely used polychrest. It has an ability to stimulate cure in a wide range of physical conditions, it helps in a crude form with the salt/fluid balance of the body and in high potency it can act as an emotional handrail helping patients to come to terms with grief and repressed buried feelings which can cause introversion, isolation and a reluctance to show emotions through fear of being seen to be vulnerable and exposed.

Dr. Cole of Albion, New York wrote that a stubborn case of urticaria had not responded to *Apis* (made from the poison of the bee sting) or *Urtica urens* (made from a variety of stinging nettle), until he progressed to the deeper acting mineral remedy of *Skookum Chuck* in just the 3x potency. The urticaria disappeared within a week. ("Homœopathic International", Spring 1994).

85

Remedies where heat is involved in the preparation of the remedy, appear to work even more deeply. The carbons, *Causticum* and *Phosphorus* come into this category. *Carbo veg* is obviously plant based, whilst *Carbo animalis* is a mineral remedy, it is no surprise that in his "Materia Medica" Phatak says of *Carbo animalis*, "More deep acting than *Carbo veg*".

All the carbons act deeply, but especially with *Carbo animalis* we see, "*Carbo animalis* is one of the deep acting, long-acting medicines. Suitable in complaints that come on insidiously, that develop slowly, that become chronic and often malignant in character. Complaints in anaemia, broken down constitutions..... We see that the economy of this patient is in a sluggish state; there are no rapid changes; but everything is slowed down..... The proving of *Carbo animalis* presents the appearance of a broken down constitution. It brought out in the provers just such symptoms as occur in old feeble constitutions, with poor repair and lack of reaction." Here we have a remedy useful for elderly people where reactive powers are slower. It is useful for very slow moving conditions, hence its reputation in helping the body under the strain of malignant conditions.

We need to emphasis the need to progress slowly to our deeper remedies. This is why, for instance, Hahnemann spoke against the use of *Phosphorus* in cases of deficient vitality and Kent suggested palliation by such a plant remedy as *Sanguinaria*. These plant remedies said Kent could build up the patient so that he could, "take a medium potency of a deep remedy" ("Lectures on Materia Medica", Kent).

The reader with a scientific background will understand the periodic table of elements and this again will enable us to compare the depth of action of certain elements. From this we know that calcium based remedies work more profoundly than magnesium based ones, and potassiums more profoundly than the sodiums.

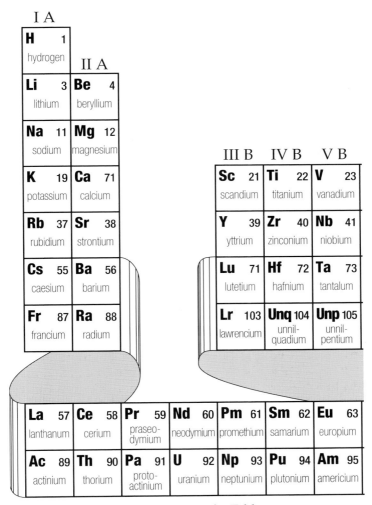

Part of the Periodic Table

Above all our aim is that this chapter should be practical and encourage the practitioner to develop a sequential form of prescribing in order to obtain the desired results. The case histories in Chapter 7 will help to illustrate this further.

CHAPTER SIX

ACUTE MENTAL CONDITIONS
("THE ORGANON" REVISITED ESPECIALLY PARAS 210 - 236)

Anyone reading this book so far would be forgiven for believing that we started every case with *Sulphur* or *Psorinum*, with the occasional exception of a dyscrasia or sycotic remedy. Conventional homœopaths, if starting with these remedies will usually do so on the basis of the symptom picture as they perceive it. They will not do so on the basis of treating first the psoric miasm.

So do we think it ever justified to start a prescription taking into account nothing but the symptom picture? We would find it difficult to hold this view based on "Chronic Diseases", but the situation can be different with certain acute conditions, especially mental conditions. By definition, "Chronic Diseases" does not try to cover these.

We are told in "The Organon" in paras 210 to 219 that if a

patient arrives for treatment with a physical condition, we take into account the state of mind and then seek a medicine from, "among the antipsoric remedies" (Para 220). Paragraph 221 of "The Organon" however is very significant:

"If, however, insanity or mania (precipitated by fright, vexation, alcohol, etc.) suddenly bursts forth as an acute disease from the patient's usually calm condition, although it almost always arises from internal psora (like a flame flaring up from it), at this initial, acute stage it should immediately be treated, not with anti-psoric remedies, but with medicines such as *Aconite, Belladonna, Stramonium, Hyoscyamus, Mercury,* etc., chosen from the other group of proved remedies and given in highly potentized subtle homœopathic doses, so as to overcome it to the point where the psora returns for the time being to its former, almost latent condition, in which the patient appears to be well."

We are told, therefore, that if we are dealing with an acute mental or emotional problem, not relating to, or derived from a physical disease, we should not immediately use *Sulphur* or *Psorinum*, although the problem almost always arises from psora. In order for the patient not to be totally overwhelmed by grief, fear, despair, schizophrenia, etc.; we do not want to dig too deep with our cleansing psoric remedies and exacerbate any symptoms in the process. A leaflet prepared by the Society of Homœopaths for new and potential patients entitled, "Homœopathy Simply Explained" states, "After taking your remedy you should notice some changes. For instance it occasionally happens that your symptoms appear worse for a short time. This is the remedy taking effect and you should feel the beginnings of recovery when this period has passed...... If you develop a runny cold, a rash or some form of discharge this will probably be the remedy having a 'spring cleaning' effect cleansing the body."

If the symptoms that get worse for a short time are connected with a skin rash, or are a mild catarrhal problem, then the patient knows that something is happening as a result of the remedies, and that a short amount of patience will be rewarded by results. However, if the symptoms are related to a suicidal despair, obviously the patient cannot tolerate any exacerbation, so here Hahnemann advises suppression. He advises choosing a remedy solely on the symptom picture in order to subdue the condition so that the psora reverts, "to its former latent state wherein the patient appears as if quite well".

Hahnemann emphasises that we have not cured the patient but that we should work to heal him completely, "by means of a prolonged anti-psoric treatment" (para 222). Moreover, he says that if this is not done, then a slighter cause than brought on the first acute attack or condition will bring on another more severe episode which will be more difficult to cure (para 223).

This line of argument is similar to that used in the first few pages of his work "Chronic Diseases", where he says the following about prescribing on cases according to the symptom picture without the use of anti-psoric treatment "Their beginning was promising, the continuation less favourable, the outcome hopeless".

We should also add, before we move on to illustrate the above, that Samuel Hahnemann also spoke of the value of counselling and psychotherapy is such cases. He used rather quaint language compared with today's, i.e. "sensible friendly exhortations, consolatory arguments, serious representations and sensible advice"; but made the point that whilst homœopathy can help as an emotional handrail, other assistance can be useful in supporting people through their difficulties.

Mr. D was a trained accountant who was unable to hold his job down when he came for treatment. He said that he felt slow, out of balance, unreal, indecisive. His brain kept 'snapping' and he felt 'black inside'. Time seemed slow and distances seemed very long. He described certain smells and tastes as being more vivid than they actually were. In the middle of a sentence he would forget what he was saying. He had a fear of the occult, having been 'sucked in' to black magic when he was at college, and considered that he heard voices telling him what to do. He was afraid that he was going mad and if homœopathy didn't work for him he planned to go and stay in a mental hospital.

He had a schizophrenic breakdown eight years previously after taking LSD and for the last year he had been regularly smoking cannabis. Cannabis has the capacity to change peoples perceptions and whatever the root of his problem there appeared to be an acute mental state brought on by a cannabis dyscrasia. The provings of *Cannabis indica* include many of the symptoms of which he complained, and accordingly he needed *Cannabis indica* in high and descending potencies.

When seen again he said that he had felt, "ten feet tall" immediately after the prescription and his confidence had improved. He was letting his emotions out now and his delusions were still there but improving all the time. He felt that his general health was better, but that he still had a long way to go before he could consider himself cured.

Mr D's condition may well have been suppressed and pushed into latency, to use Hahnemann's terminology, but he was continuing to function more and more normally. The choice now was whether to use *Sulphur* or *Psorinum*, or to leave the homœopathic prescription of *Cannabis* to work a little longer in the system.

The latter course was decided upon. Whether this was the best decision with hindsight can be argued because when seen again we had a very different story. He was totally obsessed with evil, the devil and his history of involvement in the occult. He didn't want a homœopathic remedy which might make him calmer as he needed all his strength to fight against the devil and if he lost control he felt the devil would take over. He also saw his father on occasions as the personification of the devil.

It appeared due to his past occult involvement, that he had severe spiritual problems for which he later sought help with a Christian minister, but there was a strong mental psychiatric layer on top of this which needed to be helped, again by being pushed into latency, so that he might have the faculties to seek further help. In this case he was given the remedy *Mancinella*; a single dose in the 10M homœopathic potency. It was suggested that this remedy would help him and he decided to take it as it might help in his fight against evil.

Mancinella is an uncommon remedy made from a tincture of the fruit, leaves and bark of the Manchineel tree. It has not been thoroughly proved and much of our information about it stems from the work and research of George Vitoulkas, a well-known Greek homœopath. He has done much work in studying the emotional and mental symptoms produced by homœopathic remedies by comparing the symptoms elicited in provings with the symptoms common in cured cases.

Clarke in his, "Dictionary" states that a person needing *Mancinella* has a fear of going crazy and of evil spirits. Vithoulkhas emphasises the torment of these obsessions that the person is going crazy or being taken over by the devil and that he or she needs all his or her faculties and energy to prevent this from happening. They fear that their mind is not working properly and personify any dark element as the devil. They are people lacking in self-confidence and this weakness makes them very dependent upon the people with whom they live. However there is always a dark side, a sick mind and a battle inside and often a fight between them and the devil so that they will not be taken over and possessed.

It is a remedy which we have only used three or four times in our career and the need for it has always been triggered by a horror film like, "The Exorcist" or by a bad experience with some occult type role.

With Mr D the remedy had a remarkable effect. At the next consultation he acted much more normally and never once mentioned his concern with the demonic. He appeared much more in contact with reality and perceptions and sensations were much more within the normal ranges than when he was first seen.

He expressed a feeling of loneliness and a desire to be with people all the time. He wanted to leave his father's home and get a flat for himself but was afraid of being on his own. His confidence was still at a very low ebb. He felt weak, but the major factor stopping him progressing in life appeared to be his difficulty in making the simplest decision for fear of making a mistake. He had not broken totally from his occult practices and relied on dice, horoscopes etc. to help him decide whether or not to go out in the evening or the following day.

His indecisiveness, mood changes and desire for company all pointed to the remedy *Pulsatilla*. However, we were no longer dealing with the extreme acute state of previous weeks. If we simply prescribed *Pulsatilla* then, according to what we have already described, we would soon find ourselves dispensing more and more remedies as we chased more and more symptoms. In that instance, the least trigger could have thrown him again in such another acute *Cannabis* or *Mancinella* state that he may have ended up on psychotic drugs.

This was the time to deal with those conditions which had been pushed into latency. Accordingly, *Psorinum* was needed in descending potency to be followed by *Hepar sulph* for his over sensitivity and the effect of his mercury fillings and then *Pulsatilla*. After this prescription he began to see a counsellor, found an accountancy job which he was able to hold down and felt that the remedies had helped and were continuing to help him remain stable.

It is interesting that the remedies which Hahnemann himself mentions in para 221 of "The Organon" are *Aconite, Belladonna, Stramonium, Hyoscyamus* and *Mercury*. With the exception of *Mercury* they are all alkaloid-containing plant remedies with hallucinogenic properties.

The remedy *Aconite*, or wolf's bane is used acutely for intense fear and panic, or for patients who have never been well since a fright or shock. Recent earthquakes in mid-Europe necessitated the prescribing of *Aconite* on an unprecedented scale. It is recounted that Mark Anthony's army mistook this plant for horseradish and everyone who ate of it died of heart failure, in a state of shock, with symptoms of terror, anxiety, fear and restlessness along with palpitations and tachycardia. Therefore used homœopathically, it is one of our main remedies where complaints follow fright, especially where a fear of death is involved. It has cured panic attacks which started after a fright where the person thought they would die as well as nightmares in children coming on after being frightened. It is rendered harmless and non-toxic by the homœopathic preparation of potentisation and then regularly used for states accompanied by a great fear, worry and anxiety.

Belladonna is another plant remedy, made from deadly nightshade, and which acts on every part of the nervous system. It is used homœopathically to help with symptoms which may come and go suddenly and which may include illusions, delusions and hallucinations far removed from reality. Furious rages may accompany them with an acuteness of all senses.

Stramonium, made from the thorn apple, has certain similarities both botanically and medicinally to *Belladonna*. Boericke states of *Stramonium*, "The entire force of this drug seems to be expended on the brain". Rapid changes from joy to depression and fear are common. There can be a dread of the dark and a need for light and company. Delusions about his identity as well as religious mania characterised by ceaseless talking, and occasionally by violence are common.

One patient involved in nursing was attacked by a mentally ill patient at night and after that became frightened of the dark and desired company in the evenings. Her headaches and generally feeling of well-being were improved with *Stramonium* and she then went on to require further psoric remedies.

Another patient admitted to periods of depression and also rages when she would cut herself with broken glass and wreck her flat. She could get very aggressive and attack her boyfriend with a knife. She would also easily be on the phone for an hour pouring out her troubles and needing sympathy. She had nightmares that her flat was haunted and could wake terrified. A history of being raped in her flat, a close friend being killed plus being burgled herself three times all added to the state in which she now found herself. After *Stramonium* she was sleeping better with less nightmares and feeling physically improved. Anti-psoric dyscrasia treatment was now needed in order to see her physical and mental health continue to improve.

Of the symptoms of *Hyosyamus* or henbane, Boericke says, "it is as if some diabolical force took possession of the brain and prevented its functions. It causes a perfect picture of mania of a quarrelsome and obscene character".

The above remedies will often be sufficient to help a person on the verge of a schizophrenic or psychotic breakdown and then anti-psoric treatment may be given to help the condition on a more profound level.

Mercurius being a mineral, is a remedy which will help a person on a deeper chronic level, but it can also produce and therefore cure very pronounced mental conditions. Hahnemann must have met with many people who proved mercury in its crude form. He found a feeling of panic that something was going wrong with their body or mind. The people felt that they were going insane and couldn't stand even the smallest of stresses. This is a remedy often used when a person has confronted stress after stress, (it may be bureaucracy, a family problem or a court battle) until the system breaks down.

A patient started to have panic attacks after the stress of a lengthy adoption process. *Mercurius sol* in the 200th potency helped to stabilise her, and then *Psorinum, Hepar sulph* and then *Nux vomica* in descending potencies ensured a more stable and lasting cure.

More chronic mental conditions may be dealt with immediately by miasmatic treatment because the condition has already been pushed into a latent state by homœopathic remedies, allopathic treatment or simply by the passage of time.

Therefore when Mrs B came saying that she was depressed, fed up with life, tearful, irritable, weak and comfort-eating on sweets and junk food there was no need for an acute remedy to prevent her doing anything to harm herself or others. She said that she became depressed each winter with the lack of sunlight. Accordingly she was prescribed:

Day 1	*Psorinum* 10M, 1M, 200
Day 2	*Psorinum* 30, 12, 6
Days 3 - 7	*Hepar sulph* 30 - morning
	Phos ac 30 - afternoon
	Sepia 30 - evening.

This was followed by a break of a week and then a repeat of the above prescription.

The picture of *Psorinum* includes anxiety, depression and the fact that everything is being performed in a minor key. *Hepar sulph* was given for the extreme sensitivity, as well as for any potential problems from her mercury amalgam fillings.

Both *Sepia* and *Phos acid* overlap in their ability to treat the over-riding mental state. *Sepia* works from a more hormonal angle whilst *Phos ac* being a mineral based remedy works at a deeper level and also will help more with the hypoglycaemic aspect of Mrs B's health.

A month later Mrs B said that she was 90% better and still improving. She felt better in herself, more relaxed and her energy was more normal. She also remarked that the second course had been more significant. When using descending potencies we are, to a degree, curtailing the action of the previous higher potencies. Therefore, our remedies, other than some of the deeper acting mineral remedies, can in the initial stages bear frequent repetition. Had further remedies been necessary we would have worked to eradicate from the system the toxicity caused by stress, diet and other factors as described in chapter 4.

CHAPTER SEVEN

THE PRESCRIPTION REVISITED

We have been primarily concerned in this book with chronic diseases, but it may happen that during treatment for a long standing problem the patient succumbs to an acute illness. This may be an acute flare up of a chronic condition or it may simply be what is termed a 'non-descript' virus infection. Another possibility is that it is an aggravation due to the homœopathic treatment. This may need explaining because homœopathic remedies are free from side effects, in a conventional sense, as in the method of preparation any toxic material has been removed.

However, if the body is in a state of considerable toxicity it may be stimulated to have something of a spring clean. When a room is swept for the first time the dust may fly, but the more often it is swept the less dust there is. So it is with our bodies, it is not unusual after treatment for a patient to develop a slightly runny nose for a few days, for the urine to be slightly stronger or more copious, or even for there to be a mild headache as the body is discharging toxins. Rarely will anything severe be seen, especially if the homœopath has used drainage remedies like *Berberis* to assist the liver and kidneys in their eliminative function. Homœopathic aggravations are generally a good sign as they are only transient and the patient should be in a better state of health afterwards.

Treatment of all of the above will be very similar. Firstly the practitioner will try to assess the seriousness of the condition and discuss with the patient what is happening. It will often be that reassurance is all that is required. The need for urgent investigations and casualty treatment should never be overlooked, but if the condition is considered homœopathically treatable there are simple options and steps that can be taken.

Firstly, if it appears that there is a homœopathic aggravation, and despite reassurance the patient is concerned and the condition needs alleviating, it may be sufficient just to reduce the number of tablets being taken. For instance, if the dose is three tablets and these are working very deeply, then the dose may be reduced to two tablets, or if two tablets are taken each time these may be halved. The quantity may be gradually built up again with successive prescriptions. We may also consider adding drainage remedies such as *Berberis* or even other more superficial medicines if too deep a prescription has been given.

However, if we are not dealing with an aggravation but with acute disease, then if three tablets are given daily we may ask the patient to divide these, taking one, or even half a tablet periodically during that day. This frequency of repetition is allowed for in "Chronic Diseases" ; "The only allowable exception for an immediate repetition of the same medicine is when the dose of a well selected and in every way suitable and beneficial remedy has made some beginning toward an improvement, but its action ceases too quickly, its power is too soon exhausted, and the cure does not proceed any further. This is rare in chronic diseases, but in acute diseases and in chronic diseases that rise into an acute state it is frequently the case". The acute condition quickly uses up the action of the remedy so that frequent repetition acts as a filip or stimulus to the body's energy.

A further option, if we are using descending potencies on a daily basis, is to descend them more frequently such as twice or three times a day, or even every couple of hours. Any aggravation or action by one potency will to a degree be curtailed by the next lowest potency. We may descend just that one remedy or a series of remedies.

Where the condition is very acute we may rapidly descend the remedy being taken and then prescribe for the acute ailment. Because the general health has succumbed and become susceptible to the acute infection, the vitality and possibly the condition will be improved by the use of a psoric remedy such as *Sulphur* or *Psorinum*. Then remedies working on the acute level such as *Belladonna, Aconite* and *Baptisia* may be used; either descending or a few doses of the 30th potency,. The frequency of repetition will again depend on the severity of the case with periods between tablets becoming more spaced out as the patient improves.

Where there is an acute miasm such as mumps, measles or whooping cough, the writers have invariably found good results by starting with a strong anti-psoric remedy and then alternating the indicated acute remedy be it *Belladonna* 30, *Pulsatilla* 30 or *Drosera* 30 with the appropriate nosode i.e. *Parotidinum* 30, *Morbillinum* 30 or *Pertussin* 30.

Having read the principles and methodology described so far, we would like to consolidate the knowledge with case examples where people have been cured or substantially improved. Some cases which follow are very typical of the type of patient in a normal day to day practice. Other cases are slightly more unusual but significant as they relate to conditions where improvement would be very limited or very slow if the conventional single dose of a single remedy was used.

We would not like to infer that all cases are curable. We are stating that following Hahnemann's examples and adapting them for the 20th century by such modern day researchers and homœopaths as Pritam Singh, we are able to give the body the stimulus it requires. We then, having worked towards clearing away dyscrasia and miasmatic blockages, take something of a back seat as we see what the patient's own vitality is capable of achieving.

Case 1

Sinusitis and catarrh cases are treated almost daily in a busy clinic and this case is typical. Man born September 1943. Family history of sinus problems, catarrh, asthma, throat problems, arthritis and emphysema.

30.9.92 - Sinusitis. Mucus trickles down the throat. Pressure in the ears. Allergic reaction has built up tissue in the nose causing ear ache. History of bad hay fever. Stress makes this worse. Many amalgam teeth fillings. The remedies given in descending potencies were: *Psorinum, Hepar sulph, Thuja, Rhus tox* and *Tuberculinum*. *Psorinum* was given for the psoric miasm, *Hepar sulph* for the fillings, *Thuja* for the sycosis and symptomatology along with the *Hepar sulph*. *Rhus tox* to help with the allergic nature of the problem. Allergies tend to be *Tubercular* and *Tuberculinum* will also deal with the latent psoric layer.

8.11.92 - Much better for first week or so, then went down with flu which went to throat and sinuses, however sinuses not as bad as he would have expected. Sinus problems and ears ringing for last three days. There had been a partial relapse after the flu justifying a repeat prescription of *Psorinum, Hepar sulph, Thuja, Rhus tox* and *Tuberculinum*.

15.12.92 - Was better immediately and generally felt much better. Only one sinus headache. Ears less noisy. A little mucus trickles down the throat. Whilst much of the problem was now resolved his relations had suffered from similar symptoms showing that the condition was deep seated. Accordingly deeper acting remedies produced a cure. These were *Lycopodium, Medorrhinum* and *Silica* all given in descending potencies.

At the next consultation the patient said that he had been and remained perfectly well. Note that in this case, as well as in many others, a single dose of *Syphilinum* in high potency was given during the administration of *Hepar sulph*.

Case 2

Meniere's disease is not an easy condition to treat but much progress can often be made. *China officianalis* is a remedy that has tinnitus, vertigo, deafness and all the symptoms of Meniere's disease in its picture.

Women aged 65 whose mother and brother have Meniere's disease and deafness. Sister has had tuberculosis.

24.4.91 - Meniere's first appeared at age 27. Ear blocked. Pressure feeling. Pulsating, hissing. Like being in a lift. Hearing distorted. Cannot tolerate noise. Stress aggravates. Blood pressure 180/90. Remedies given in descending potencies: *Psorinum, Hepar sulph, China,* Followed by *Hepar sulph* 30 in the morning and *China* 30 in the evening for seven days.

30.5.91 - Felt the "best for six years". Coping better. Hearing better with improvement within the first two or three days. Blocked feeling gone. Pressure and pulsation gone. Tinnitus 50% improvement. Tolerating noise better. Same prescription as previous month given. By using descending potencies we are, to a degree, curtailing the action of the previous higher potency before its action has necessarily been exhausted. This means that many of our prescriptions bear repetition well, unless we are using our deepest remedies.

11.7.91 - Sleep better, the best since children were young. No bad patch. Blood pressure 162/85. Improvement maintained. She is continuing to do well, however as the condition is inherited we need to use relevant nosodes and then deeper remedies. Remedies used are *Psorinum, Hepar sulph, China, Tuberculinum* in descending potencies as before followed by 7 days of *Hepar sulph* 30 in the mornings and *China* 30 in the evenings.

1.8.91 - Blood Pressure 130/70

3.9.91 - Again felt better in self. Whilst progress has been very good there is an antidotal relationship between *China* and *Hepar sulph. Thuja* will therefore come between the two this time helping *China* to work better as well as dealing the the sycotic nature of the case. Hence the remedies: *Psorinum, Hepar sulph, Thuja, China, Tuberculinum* were given in descending potencies.

11.11.91 - Very good. A little worse since the remedies finished. *Syphilinum* is now added as a deeper acting nosode, as well as helping the body to deal as best it can with the destructive nature of Meniere's disease. Remedies - *Psorinum, Hepar sulph, Thuja, China, Syphilinum.*

18.2.91 - Fine while taking the remedies then became deafer

with pressure feeling, pulsation, hissing and roaring bad. However she then improved again, "Shortest relapse ever and delighted with the result". Deeper remedies were now given - *China, Medorrhinum, Conium, Silica* and then *Carbo animalis* all descending potencies followed by *China* 30 once a day for 10 days.

29.7.92 - "No bad spells which is fantastic. Cannot believe it can carry on like this". Blood pressure 145/88. No remedies were given.

The patient has continued to do well. *Conium* was used not only for its depth of action but also for its pace of action. It corresponds to conditions like Meniere's disease which tend to come on very slowly and similarly improves very slowly as well as covering the symptomatology of the condition. *Silica* and *Carbo animalis* continued to complement the action of the other remedies and took them into greater depth. The patient has remained relatively well.

Excessive use of Aspirin is one of the causes of ringing in the ears. Salicylic acid is the active ingredient and other cases of Meniere's disease have been considerably helped by *Salicylic acid* in potency as well as by drainage remedies such as *Berberis*.

Case 3

Pre-menstrual tension and menstrual cramp is another commonly met condition during a busy practice.

3.5.92 - Woman born May 1974. Bad period pains since age 14. First day of flow worse. Tense, irritable, tearful and wants to be on own before menses. Sore throats before periods, short cycle of 24 days.

Remedies given in descending potencies: *Psorinum, Hepar sulph, Nux vomica, Sepia* and *Tuberculinum*.

The well respected homœopath Dr. Guernsey has written that *Nux vomica* precedes *Sepia* well and will often help it to work more effectively. *Nux vomica* helped the spasmodic pains and then *Sepia* continued its work, acting on a more hormonal level.

15.5.92 - Cycle normal length. No PMT for the first time in memory. No sore throat before period which was unusual. Pain improved 30% in the abdomen but the normal drawing pain had totally gone. Finished remedies yesterday. The

Chapter 7

course of remedies was extended by *Carbo veg* followed by a
seven day gap. Remedies were then continued with
Psorinum, Hepar sulph, Nux vomica and *Sepia* given again in
descending potencies.
Carbo veg, as well as being a digestive remedy for which it is
best known, will often complete the action of *Sepia*. A week's
gap was then given before repeating the course. As further
courses are given and deeper longer lasting remedies are used,
so the lengths of the gaps between courses is correspondingly
increased.
24.6.92 - Cycle 28 days. No PMT. Heavy flow still., Bad pain
first night but for shorter duration than before. Sore throat
very slightly. Remedies extended into depth with
Tuberculinum, Lycopodium, Carbo veg and lastly *Silica*.
28.8.92 - Last period really good. No PMT and very little pain.
No sore throat. Flow less heavy. 28 day cycle. No remedy
given.
As our patient had bad pain from the onset of her periods it is
likely that there was an inherited aspect and this was dealt
with the *Silica*. *Silica* is a deep acting remedy as well as being a
large enough polycrest to cover all her troublesome symptoms.

Case 4
We would not wish to infer that sickle cell anaemia is necessarily curable with homœopathic remedies, but we can say that
this man has remained symptom free for two years after he was
last tested.
West Indian man born March 1966. Heart conditions in
family background.
15.7.91 - Tired. Joint pains. Picks up infections easily with his
condition. Pains are worse after exertion. Pains disappear as
he loosens up with gentle movement. Knee joint can be stiff.
Heat improves and cold aggravates symptoms. Has flushes
of heat. Is a born worrier and stress aggravates. Has many
amalgam tooth fillings.
Remedies given: *Psorinum, Hepar sulph, Rhus tox.
Tuberculinum* in descending potencies followed by *Hepar
sulph* 30 in the mornings and *Rhus tox* 30 in the evenings for
7 days.
Rhus tox was given for the joint pains and *Tuberculinum* for

102

the Tubercular and multi-miasmatic background.

10.9.91 - Less tired than usual. No joint pains. No flushes of heat. Feels better in himself. Remedies given *Psorinum, Hepar sulph, Thuja, Rhus tox* and *Tuberculinum. Thuja* was given for the background of sycosis, vaccination and because it precedes *Tuberculinum* well increasing its effectiveness.

26.11.91 - Finished remedies a month ago and then in hospital for two days with a crisis and severe pains. Tiredness improved since first seen. Knee joint not stiff now but can click. As he works in a hospital had a polio, hepatitis and tetanus vaccination last week. Colour of eyes less yellow. Remedies given *Psorinum, Hepar sulph, Thuja, Ferrum phos* and *Syphilinum.*

Leaving the aches and pains of *Rhus tox* we are now using the deeper mineral based remedy of *Ferrum phosphate* which works on the bloods cells themselves. *Syphilinum* is used as the conditions is characterised by the malfunction of the red blood cells related to the destructive miasma.

4.2.92 - Fine on course of remedies. Two weeks later felt tired but not as much as previously. No aches, pains or stiffness. Eyes still less yellow. Remedies given: *Psorinum, Hepar sulph, Thuja, Ferrum phos* and *Syphilinum* in descending potencies.

31.3.92 - Generally fine. Not tired. Finished remedies three weeks ago. No aches, pains or stiffness. 90% better. Remedies: nil for four weeks then *Psorinum, Hepar sulph, Ferrum phos, Medorrhinum* and *Carbo animalis.*

The heart conditions in the family background call for *Medorrhinum. Carbo animalis* is a very deep remedy suitable for cases having a destructive element being made, as it is, from destroyed animal tissue.

20.8.92 - Fine. No remedies given.

Case 5

Children with asthma, eczema and allergic conditions are seen commonly in the consulting room. Most allergies have a tubercular root, making *Psorinum* and *Tuberculinum* the prime nosodes. *Rhus tox* and *Pulstailla* are the most commonly used remedies. *Arsenicum* shares the symptomatology of *Rhus tox* but has much more anxiety and worry about their health and their security. *Arsenicum* is a profound remedy and one which in the case below did not need to be taken into greater depth with such remedies as *Silica*. Had there been any relapse of the asthma then other nosodes, drainage remedies and deeper remedies would be used.

15.5.91 - Boy born September 1982. Uncle and grandfather had asthmatic problems. Patient had an asthma attack six months after his father died of cancer. Since then he has been wheezy with a deep hoarse cough. He worries and gets very anxious about the health of his mother if she gets a cold, etc. He gets more wheezy with worry. Remedies given: *Psorinum, Arsenicum, Tuberculinum* in descending potencies, followed by *Arsenicum* 30 for 5 days.

1.7.91 - A lot better. Not so out of breath with either damp or exercise. Very little cough and not worrying so much. For the first two weeks slightly worse with skin blotches which then began to improve. Remedies given: *Psorinum, Arsenicum, Tuberculinum* in descending potencies, followed by *Arsenicum* 30 for 5 days.

There had been the not unusual 'spring cleaning' effect from the initial prescription and then improvement. There was no reason to change the prescription which was repeated after a brief interval.

11.7.91 - A phone call a week later pointed to more 'spring cleaning', ie bad nose bleed on the first day of the remedy. Very emotional recently. Worrying a lot about something happening to his mother. Leg numb. Giddy. Asthma better. Worries that if something happens to his mum he will be on his own.

This was probably all due to a mineral remedy being used as the indicated remedy. This therefore worked deeply with the effect of eradicating many impurities from the system.

Remedy: continue with the course of treatment.

2.8.91 - No asthma. More confident. Worrying less. Sleeping well. No remedy.

Case 6

Eczema case - Girl born March 1990. History of Tuberculosis, eczema and psoriasis in the family.

23.3.94 - She has had eczema for 3 months. Dry. Hot baths

aggravate. Changeable moods. Very sensitive. General health good. History of multi-vitamins and minerals.

Remedies given: *Radium bromide* descending over two days. Days 3 - 7 *Calc carb* 30, *Berberis* 30 and *Rhus tox* 30. One week with no remedies and then *Psorinum* descending over two days was given followed by *Radium bromide* 30, *Kali phos* 30 and *Pulsatilla* 30 for 5 days.

Radium bromide was given as it not only corresponds to many of the symptoms of eczema but it will also help with a system that has been overloaded with calcium and magnesium.

29.4.94 - Has had chickenpox but exceptionally mildly compared to other members of the family. Eczema has gone as has the itching leaving just a little dry skin. Much better before second course started. No need of any more treatment at present. No remedies needed but *Psorinum* descending over two days followed by five days of *Hepar sulph* 30, *Kali phos* 30 and *Rhus tox* 30 were given to hold in case symptoms return. We would consider *Tuberculinum* if further treatment is needed.

Case 7

Chemically related eczema case; an who works a lot with cleaning fluids.

20.5.94 - Dry skin on hands could be chemically related. Spots and vesicles under the skin which weep and discharge clear fluid. Itches and feels stiff. Water aggravates as do chemicals. The right hand is worse. Started four years ago on one finger. Last three months has got worse. Stress makes no difference. Is generally better in the wind, perspires a lot and is worse for heat.

Remedies given: *Psorinum* descending over two days. Days 3 - 7 *Radium Bromide* 30, *Berberis* 30 and *Rhus tox* 30 each day. One weeks break followed by *Sulphur* descending over two days followed by *Hepar sulph* 30, *Kali phos* 30 and *Rhus tox* 30 for the next five days.

23.6.94 - Started to improve during the first week and then got worse. Skin is less weepy, there are fewer large spots. It has been more itchy in the last few days with stiffness and worse for heat.

Remedies given: *Radium bromide* descending over two days followed by *Thuja* 30, *Echinacea* 30 and *Rhus tox* 30 over the following five days. Two weeks break followed by *Tuberculinum* descending over two days followed by *Radium bromide* 30, *Kali phos* 30 and *Lycopodium* 30.

20.7.94 - Cancelled appointment as hands perfect.

Case 8

Migraine case of a woman born February 1949. Her father and mother both have high blood pressure. Her mother and mother's grandfather suffered migraine.

23.2.93 - Frequent migraines related to relief of stress after meeting deadlines. Gets a 'detached' feeling, vomits and wants dark and quiet. Generally catarrhal. Affected by stress. Needs to be in control and does not delegate.

Remedies given sequentially in descending potencies: *Psorinum, Hepar sulph, Thuja* and *Arsenicum album.*

Again the anxiety when not in control calls for *Arsenicum. Arsenicum* works more effectively following *Thuja.* Most importantly *Arsenicum* is antidoted by *Hepar sulph* and therefore should not follow it directly. Also it is best not to have two mineral based remedies next to each other but where possible to have a plant based remedy in between.

26.3.93 - Had two migraines which have been less intense and shorter than normal. Didn't vomit and detached feeling was less. More catarrh that usual at first. The 'spring cleaning' effect meant that the body was working to eradicate toxins and that the prescription could be repeated to advantage. Hence the remedies given were: *Psorinum, Hepar sulph, Thuja, Arsenicum album* and then *Tuberculinum* all sequential and in descending potencies. The addition of *Tuberculinum* allowed the prescription to work deeper in the areas of latent psora.

19.5.93 - 'Mini' migraine on third day and since then nothing. Still some catarrh in the background. Remedies given in the same way were *Lycopodium* and *Wiersbaden.* With migraine in the family background it was considered that using deeper acting remedies would afffect the inherited predisposition and work towards preventing a relapse.

26.7.93 No migraine. Best for over three years. Always a background of catarrh. Remedies given *Psorinum* descending in two days followed by *Hepar sulph* 30, *Berberis* 30 and *Natrum sulph* 30 for five days. *Natrum sulph* is a deeper sycotic remedy than *Thuja*, dealing with the catarrh. Also using *Berberis* as a drainage remedy would help the kidneys to eradicate more effectively the body's toxic load.

26.10.93 - No migraines and not troubled by catarrh. No remedies given.

Case 9

Fibroid case - Many consider that fibroid problems can only be dealt with by surgery, however with homœopathy we often see the fibroid shrink or at least the symptoms resolve. This women was born in February 1950 and there was a family history of cancer, tuberculosis and heart attacks.

2.9.92 - General continual ache with fibroids all the time in the abdomen. Heartburn for 18 months. Periods heavier and now only 14 days apart. Tired. Premenstually very intolerant. Many amalgam tooth fillings. Hair loss.

The following remedies were given sequentially in descending potencies. *Psorinum, Hepar sulph, Thuja* and *Tuberculinum*.

Fibroids are obviously related to the sycotic maism. The Greek homœopath George Vithoulkas says that he never uses Thuja in cases of fibroids as they can get larger. However to use descending potencies channels the action of the remedies providing a vent at a physical and pathological level. Hence we are controlling the action of our remedies obtaining results and preventing undesirable side effects.

13.10.92 - No pain for one week, then it returned but not so badly. Heartburn is rare now. Last period much better and only lasted seven days. Pain only lasted twelve hours which is "remarkable - best I can remember". Energy much improved. Co-ordination better. PMT improved. Itchiness and cramp gone. Hair loss still same.

Remedies given in descending potencies: *Psorinum, Hepar sulph, Thuja, Medorrhinum* and *Phytolacca. Medorrhinum* is the main sycotic nosode and *Phytolacca*, although a plant remedy, being made from the root, is a relatively deep acting fibroid medicine.

10.12.92 - Stomach fine. No heartburn. PMT considerable less. Fibroid ache improved 80%. Better sustained energy. Last period much more normal. Remedies given were again *Psorinum, Hepar sulph, Thuja, Medorrhinum, Phytolacca.*

26.1.93 - No pain or bleeding or any indications of having a fibroid. Hair loss improved. Periods excellent. No PMT. Remedies given *Conium* and *Wiersbaden.* Fibroids grow slowly. *Conium* is a remedy for slow moving conditions including growths, tumours, etc. *Wiersbaden* is a remedy produced from a mineral rich Prussian spring water. It is therefore a multi-mineral remedy in its own right bringing such remedies as *Thuja* and *Conium* into greater depth. the symptom picture of *Wiersbaden* has hair loss as a pronounced feature.

9.4.93 - Had flu but fully recovered. No problems. No remedies required.

Case 10
Endometriosis case. Women born May 1967. Grandparents and parents had kidney problems and mother was on drugs for such problems during conception. Mother, sister and two cousins had painful periods.

24.2.93 - Patient had ovarian cyst removed and endometriosis started after the operation. Periods are now always heavy with intermittent bleeding. More painful at ovulation and period time. All periods are equally bad. Tiredness, backache, PMT and fluid retention with periods. Remedies given sequentially and in descending potencies: *Psorinum, Hepar sulph, Thuja* and *Sepia.* Endometriosis relates more to the sycotic miasm, hence the use of *Thuja*, whilst *Sepia* relates to much of the hormonal symptomatolgy.

30.3.93 - "On top of the world". Period shorter than normal and more normal period pain. No tiredness. Back to old self. PMT lasted a day instead of a week. Remedies given were *Psorinum, Hepar sulph, Thuja, Sepia* and *Tuberculinum* in the same way.

4.5.93 - Period a better colour. Felt healthier. Period heavy but for a short time. Not painful at ovulation. "The difference between existing and living". Craves sweet things before periods. Remedies given: *Phos ac, Lycopodium, Medorrhinum,*

Carbo veg. With painful periods in the family background it was necessary to use deeper remedies as well as *Medorrhinum* being the main sycotic nosode.

5.7.93 - A few stress headaches. Feels better within self. Ovulation pain shorter. Remedies given: *Psorinum* descending in two days followed by *Hepar sulph* 30, *Nux vomica* 30 and *Sepia* 30 for five days.

10.11.93 - Periods fine and energy good. Pain for eight days with stress of emotions from break up of a relationship. Remedies: *Psorinum* descending in two days followed by *Hepar sulph* 30, *Nux vomica* 30 and *Sepia* 30 for five days.

22.12.93 - No ovulation pain or headaches. No period pains or PMT. Fine.

Case 11

Osteo -arthritis case. This is a condition rarely helped by conventional homeopathy but the following two cases illustrate the benefit of this form of treatment when the patient has a good vitality and the condition is not too advanced.

Case of a woman born February 1938 with arthritis in the family background.

2.3.93 - Osteo-arthritis in both hips, started 15 - 20 years ago. Stiff in morning, loosens up later but no change in pain. Warmth ameliorates. Had many amalgam fillings in teeth. Remedies given sequentially and in descending potencies: *Psorinum, Hepar sulph, Symphytum, Tuberculinum, Ledum.*

10.4.93 - Stiffness improved slightly. Very little change. Remedies given in the same way: *Psorinum, Hepar sulph, Symphytum, Syphilinum, Lycopodium.*

17.5.93 - Telephone call - pain had increased substantially and the patient was very despondent. Patient was given the reassurance that something was happening as a result of the stimulus her body had received from the remedies.

28.5.93 - Nails growing quicker! Obviously growth has been stimulated. More pain in hip but walking better and not needing to take pain killers at night now. Stiffness less. We continued with deeper acting remedies: *Psorinum, Silica* and *Carbo animalis.*

21.7.93 - Much better than when first seen. Still making progress and people say she looks better. There is less pain in her hips and she can stand and walk for longer. Nails still growing amazingly quickly. No remedy was given and the patient continued to make good progress.

Case 12

Osteo-arthritis Case. Woman born February 1946. Family history of heart problems, depression and cancer with arthritis on her father's side.

30.8.93 - Pain began in the spring four years ago following a fall and got worse recently. Fatigue. Lethargy. Stiffness of all joints. Damp and cold makes it worse. Much catarrh. Ache back of neck and slight headache. Skin rashes. Remedies given sequentially and in descending potencies: *Psorinum, Hepar sulph, Berberis, Rhus tox* and *Tuberculinum*. Although osteo-arthritis would normally call for such remedies as *Symphytum*, theses symptoms corresponded very much to the provings of *Rhus tox*. *Arnica* (the pre-eminent first-aid, bruise remedy) could have been given for the history of the fall but the remedies given proved this unnecessary.

30.9.93 - "50% improved". Less fatigue. No headaches. Not so hungry. More well being. Kidneys more efficient. Stiffness a lot better. Some hand joint pain which was a return of old symptoms, which the body had not properly dealt with in the past and which showed a progression on the road to cure. Skin eruption gradually lessened. Back of neck much improved. Cold weather not making the same difference. Remedies given in the same way: *Lycopodium, Silica, Carbo animalis*.

Osteo-arthritis is a serious degenerative condition which is not going to be thoroughly dealt with without our deepest mineral remedies, especially when the condition is also in the family background.

12.11.93 - Better in self. Emotionally clearer in mind. Not having bouts of depression. A few spots, nodules came and went. Increase in bowel and bladder functions. Great improvement in lower part of the spine. Joint pains gone. Remedies given: *Radium bromide* descending over three days, followed by *Radium bromide* 30, *Symphytum* 30 and *Ledum* 30 for five days. We are now building on the foundations we have laid with our deep acting remedies.

11.12.93 - Joint pains and spine good. No pains. Skin good now. Liver fine. Bowels and urine fine. Much better generally. Remedies given: *Psorinum* descending over three days followed by *Hepar sulph* 30, *Taraxacum* 30 and *Symphytum* 30 for five days.

20.2.94 - "Wonderfully well". Working longer hours. Sleeping well. No pain. Looser in movements. Energy much better. Not depressed. Skin fine.

Case 13

Snoring Case - Man born June 1931. Relatives had asthma, bronchitis and nasal polyps. Father snored badly.

18.11.92 - Radioactive burn out of thyroid gland one year ago and on thyroxin since March. Snoring much of late, breathing stops then he wakes. Sneezing with sunlight. Fatigue and irritability. Many teeth fillings over the years. Remedies given sequentially and in descending order: *Psorinum Hepar sulph, Opium, Tuberculinum* and *Radium bromide*. *Opium*, as a poison, is known for producing snoring and stertorous breathing. It is not a remedy we use often but it has a place as a more superficial remedy. The history of radioactive treatment pointed to the use of *Radium bromide* in potency.

6.1.93 - Sweating at night has disappeared, twitching gone, snoring slightly better. Still sneezes in sunlight. Remedies given in same way: *Lycopodium, Syphilinum, Silica*. The family history pointed towards the need for deeper acting remedies covering the symptomatology.

8.3.93 - Telephone to cancel appointment as all symptoms better.

Case 14

This is a case of a man aged 34 whose father suffered from indigestion and he had permanent indigestion. He takes Rennies indigestion tablets persistently. Has had a barium meal X-ray and a small hiatus hernia was diagnosed. Stomach producing too much acid. Fats aggravate. Has had indigestion every day for two years. Acid in oesophagus causing burning pain. History of indigestion as child. Drinks 10 pints of beer a week.

6.3.94 - Remedies given *Radium bromide* descending over two days followed by *Radium bromide* 30, *Berberis* 30 and *Nux vomica* 30 for five days. One week no medication and then *Psorinum* descending over two days followed by *Hepar sulph* 30, *Kali phos* 30 and *Nux vomica* 30 for five days.

The case was started with *Radium bromide* rather than *Psorinum* as the dyscrasia from the *Magnesium* and *Barium* might have been so pronounced that *Psorinum* may have been ineffective if used initially.

4.5.94 - Telephoned to report no need of ant-acids and no longer any problems.

Case 15
Irritable bowel syndrome, Hiatus hernia and stomach ulcer. Man born September 1943. Relatives had Parkinson's disease, bowel cancer, stomach cancer, constipation and arthritis.

5.3.92 - All food gives indigestion. Tagamet for eight years. Burning, burping, acid pain, distension, piles and constipation. Bottles up stress and feels angry and irritable inside. Needs to wait 4 - 5 hours to digest food before he can go to sleep and needs black coffee to get going in the morning.
Remedies given daily in descending potencies: *Psorinum, Hepar sulph, Nux vomica, Tuberculinum* followed by seven days of *Hepar sulph* 30 in the morning and *Nux vomica* 30 in the evening.

16.4.92 - Slightly better. 20% better. Some days can go without Tagamet. Not all food gives indigestion now and feels easier in self. Remedies again given daily in descending potency: *Radium bromide, Hepar sulph, Nux vomica, Tuberculinum, Lycopodium.*

2.6.92 - 40% better. Generally on an upward curve. Tagamet about twice weekly now. Remedies given in descending potencies: *Psorinum, Carbo veg, Podophyllum* and *Silica.* These are the deeper acting remedies which have an affinity for the digestive area.

10.8.92 - Stopped Tagamet a month ago. Digestion not a problem and stomach and bowels are fine. Not troubled by constipation or piles. Energy improved. Again the problem is apparently sorted out by the use of remedies working deeper in the system. No remedies given.

Case 16
Prostate problems. Man born October 1933 presented with increasing prostate problems over the last ten years. Passed small amount of blood in urine a year ago. Aggravated by cold weather. Much dental work including amalgam fillings twenty years ago. Some abdominal wind.

Remedies given in descending potencies daily: *Psorinum, Hepar sulph, Thuja, Tuberculinum* and *Sabal serrulata. Thuja* covers the symptomatology of prostate problems, though the main remedy is *Sabal serrulata* made from the Saw palmetto berry.

5.11.93 - Great improvement. Gets up to urinate 2-3 times each night whereas it used to be 5-6 times. He had noticed a lot of improvement on the *Hepar sulph.* No problems during the day now. Felt he was 70% improved but had no change in abdominal wind. Remedies given: *Lycopodium, Conium* and *Silica.*

It would have been justified to repeat the original prescription but as the condition was both inherited and long standing for ten years it was decided to use deeper remedies covering the symptomolgy. *Conium* also covers the pace, i.e. slow development of the condition.

29.12.93 - Improvement maintained. Some improvement in abdominal wind. Had a past history of many antacids. The feeling that the bladder does not empty completely has improved recently. Remedies: *Radium bromide* descending over three days followed by *Hepar sulph* 30, *Berberis* 30 and *Sabal serrulata* 30 for five days. Fourteen days with no remedies followed by *Medorrhinum* descending over three days followed by *Thuja* 30, *Taraxacum* 30 and *Sabal serullata* 30 for five days.

Radium bromide was given to deal with the antacid/magnesium dyscrasia which had recently come to light. Also drainage remedies were now given to aid the elimination of the system.

12.2.94 - Fine in the day and some improvement in some nights. Wind improved greatly. Still some tightness in prostate - does not always feel relaxed. The following short courses were given, one each month for the next three months.

February - *Sulphur* descending over four days followed by *Thuja* 30, *Kali phos* 30 and *Conium* 30 for five days.

March - *Kali phos* descending over four days followed by *Natrum sulph* 30, *Kali phos* 30 and *Sabal Serrulata* 30 for 5 days.

April - *Causticum* descending over four days followed by *Hepar sulph* 30, *Causticum* 30 and *Conium* 30 for five days.

It was decided to alternate *Sabal Serrulata* and *Conium* in the 30th potency for the prostate gland as well as using progressively deeper acting drainage remedies (see Chapter 4). *Sulphur* was used as an alternative to *Psorinum* as it better covered the symptoms of his condition.

28.4.94 - Nights a lot better now. Generally up once a night only now and some nights not at all. It had been a gradual improvement. Tightness no longer a problem and his stomach was fine.

May - *Psorinum* descending over three days followed by *Thuja* 30, *Berberis* 30 and *Sabal serrlata* 30.

June - *Tuberculinum* descending over three days followed by *Hepar sulph* 30, *Berberis* 30 and *Conium* 30 for five days.

No further treatment was necessary.

Case 17

Glue ear problems are becoming more common. This girl came at two and a half years old.

26.6.94 - Ear infections every time she teethes. She had been screaming with pain the previous night with a temperature. Hearing appears normal on some days and down on others. Colds normally go to the ears. Off food and drink when ears bad. Temperature 102 deg. Left ear red.

Remedies: *Psorinum* descending followed quickly by *Pulsatilla* descending followed by *Calc carb* 30, *Berberis* 30 and *Pulsatilla* 30. One week gap followed by *Radium bromide* descending over two days followed by *Radium bromide* 30, *Kali phos* 30 and *Thuja* 30 for five days.

The first course sorted out the ear problem and she had been consistently well since then. Had there been any further problem *Tuberculinum* would have been used but three months later she still needed no further treatment.

Case 18

Thrush and varicose veins. Woman born 8.11.59, both parents had varicose veins. Mother also had angina and the father high blood pressure. Maternal grandmother died from heart disease. 12.4.94 - Continual vaginal thrush since January; itching, sore skin with cracks and a white discharge. Varicose veins which started during her second pregnancy. She has two children aged 6 and 4 years. Pain comes and goes. Vein in her left leg 'blew up' last November. She had been given *Arnica* and *Hamamelis* for three months from another clinic with no improvement. Movings and pulsating in the legs with twitching. Deep aching in the leg and in the thigh. Varicose veins worse in the left leg and incompetent veins in both legs. Feet always cold. Legs feel better after a hot bath. Remedies: *Psorinum* descending over two days followed by *Hepar sulph* 30, *Berberis* 30 and *Pulsatilla* 30 for 5 days. One week free followed by *Radium bromide* descending over two days and then *Radium bromide* 30, *Kali phos* 30 and *Pulsatilla* 30 for five days.

Pulsatilla is being used for her condition; it covers both the symptoms of the thrush and the varicose veins. To ease pressure on the veins, drainage remedies were introduced early on to help the body to filter out its toxic load.

13.5.94 -Immediate relief with legs at start of the remedies. However after finishing the first course the pain came back straight away. Started next course on Friday, three days early. Felt fine while standing for a long period at an exhibition. Not a constant ache now and "not living with it all the time. Two- thirds improved". Feet still cold. Thrush has gone. Remedies given: *Psorinum* descending over two days followed by *Hepar sulph* 30, *Kali phos* 30 and *Pulsatilla* 30 for five days. Two weeks with no remedies and then given *Kali phos* descending over two days followed by *Folliculinum* 30, *Kali phos* 30 and *Pulsatilla* 30 for five days.

By September 1994 there had been no return of the thrush and the varicose veins were much improved. For future treatment, possibilities would be to progress from *Kali phos* to the deeper drainage remedy of *Causticum* and also to use the indicated remedies in descending potencies progressing to the deeper mineral based remedies such as *Silica*.

Case 19

Depression, arthritis and shingles. Woman born July 1918. Sister also has arthritis and depression.

17.12.92. - Clinical depression. No energy. Sits for hours staring into space. A worrier. Memory is poor. Apathy is getting worse, life is a struggle. The arthritis is in the knees dating back to a fall twenty years ago. The bone is very worn and this affects her back. Wet, damp aggravates. She has had shingles for six months on back and chest which came on after the worry of moving house.

Remedies given in descending potencies: *Psorinum, Hepar sulph, Phos ac* and *Tuberculinum. Phos ac* is a remedy for the effects of either shocks and griefs or life's struggles leading to apathy and lethargy.

14.1.93 - Stopped anti-depressants. Hands steady. Apathy and depression are gone. Shingles has improved substantially although under the arms is still painful, like ants biting. Legs are very swollen and heavy and knees are painful.

Remedies given in descending potencies: *Rhus tox, Symphytum, Ledum* and *Lycopodium. Rhus tox* covers the symptoms of both shingles and rheumatism. *Symphytum* will help to build up bone tissue and *Ledum* has *Rhus tox* symptoms with bone changes.

18.2.93 - Depression and apathy not returned. Shingles are no longer painful, though tender and sore. Legs not swollen and not as heavy. Pain in left knee improved. Pain in right knee is still bad.

Remedies given in descending potencies: *Rhus tox, Conium, Syphilinum* and *Wiersbaden. Rhus tox*, being a key plant remedy was repeated. The wear and tear of tissue relates to the syphilitic miasm.

22.4.93 - Very well and much improved. Leg joint badly worn but walks faster and without a stick. All swelling gone as has the heavy feeling. Eating better. Left knee fine and pain in right knee much better. Has been two weeks without tablets and without problems.

This case is unusual in that one extending prescription was all that was needed. It also differed from the norm for the first indicated remedy to be mineral based. If a condition is very acute then the body's vital energy will use up the full potency of the medicine so that nothing is left to continue working at the inherited levels. This is why, as an example, *Silica* can be used acutely for abscesses because the potency is virtually all used up dealing with the acute condition.

Case 20

This is a complex case of mixed connective tissue disease and one that shows that having a strategy and using the basic homœopathic medicines brings results. The patient was a woman born July 1956. Familiy history of cancer, ovarian cysts, diverticulitis, sinusitis, hay-fever, osteo-arthritis, migraine, alcoholism and tuberculosis.

21.9.91 - Systemic lupus, tissue disease. Affects swallowing - constriction in the throat, food gets stuck in oesophagus. Tired. Tissue around joints swells and puffs up, stiff muscles with aching. Skin rashes, wheals, butterfly rash on face. Headaches, giddiness. Constipation alternating with diarrhoea. Problems started four months before marriage and are worse from stress. Many fillings.

Remedies given in descending potencies: *Psorinum, Hepar sulph, Rhus tox, Tuberculinum* followed by *Hepar sulph* 30 and *Rhus tox* 30 each day for seven days.

8.11.91 Worse on the remedies for one day then saw an improvement in the following areas - energy, dry mouth, breathlessness, PMT, headaches, tiredness, stiffness, muscle aches, giddiness, skin irritation, constipation and diarrhoea. No change in swallowing or swelling around joints. Moods and tiredness show the biggest improvement.

Remedies given again in descending potencies: *Psorinum, Hepar sulph, Thuja, Rhus tox, Tuberculinum.*

9..1.92 - Generally slight further improvement. A slight rash came and went. No change in throat spasms; as if choking. More emotionally up and down since finishing the prescription.

Remedies given in descending potencies *Psorinum, Hepar sulph, Ignatia, Syphillinum, Rhus tox. Ignatia* is a superficial acute remedy often used for emotional conditions but one which covers all the throat spasms.

16.3.92 - Kept well. Generally feels good and calmer. Throat improved.

Remedies given: *Psorinum, Hepar sulph, Rhus tox, Medorrhinum, Lycopodium.*

3.6.92 - No joint pains. Throat further improved. Energy and emotions good, had a slight skin rash. Remedies given: *Psorinum, Conium, Carbo veg* and *Silica.* Before proceeding into depth *Psorinum* was repeated to cope with the skin rash that had appeared since the last course had finished.

12.8.92 - Feeling very well. No symptoms. Finished remedies four weeks ago. Previously symptoms have reappeared since completing previous courses but not this time. No remedies given.

Case 21

Girl born June 1984. Bed wetting and arthritis are in the family background.

19.12.92 - Bed wetting twice weekly over the last four years. Sleeps deeply and wets the bed within two hours. Highly strung, nervous, shy. Urine PH 7.5 with protein trace. Has had two teeth fillings six months and two years ago.

Remedies given in descending potencies: *Psorinum, Hepar sulph, Pulsatilla, Tuberculinum, Hepar sulph* 30 and *Petroleum* 30 for five days.

4.2.93 - Urine PH 6.5. Very slight protein trace. Bed wet twice weekly still. Remedies given: *Psorinum, Hepar sulph, Thuja, Pulsatilla* and *Syphilinum.*

31.3.93 - Wet bed weekly on course; more frequently since the course of remedies had finished. Urine PH 7.5. Remedies given: *Psorinum, Hepar sulph, Pulsatilla, Tuberculinum* and *Lycopodium.*

20.5.93 - Bet wetting improved; about once a week now. Urine NAD. Remedies given: *Carbo veg* and *Silica.*

27.8.93 - Apart from a week on holiday when excited and tired is now consistently dry at night. No remedies given.

Again the case illustrates the importance of our deeper mineral based remedies.

Case 22

Gall stone colic. Woman born October 1948. Sister and an aunt with gall bladder problems, father and grandfather both had tuberculosis. Psoriasis, kidney infections, diabetes, cancer, heart trouble, arthritis and mental illness in immediate family.

21.9.92 - Gall bladder chronically contracts on a few pieces of stone giving nausea, bad indigestion, shooting pains and numbness. Also suffers from cramp, pins and needles, catarrh. Skin always icy cold. Remedies given in descending potencies of: *Psorinum, Hepar sulph, Rhus tox, Tuberculinum, Nux vomica* and *Lycopodium*.

7.11.92 - Numbness shifted to left. Burning now rather than numb. Return of old symptoms of itching and slight cystitis from two years old. Digestion fine. Cold icy feeling of skin improved. Occasional gall bladder pain. Energy better. Remedies given in descending potency: *Psorinum, Hepar sulph, Thuja, Syphilinum*.

17.12.92 - Numbness all gone. Gall bladder trouble nearly gone. Nausea less. Dealing with stress better. Thrush which was an old symptom came and went. Energy good. Remedies given: *Lycopodium, Carbo veg* and *Wiersbaden*.

13.1.93 - Telephone call: gall bladder problems worse, (may be 'spring cleaning' from deeper remedies).

4.2.93 - Gall bladder still worse. Digging in back. Thick yellow coated tongue. Finished course of remedies three weeks ago. Remedies given: *Psorinum, Hepar sulph, Berberis, Tuberculinum, Lycopodium, Silica. Psorinum* was given here to stimulate the immune system. *Berberis* was added as a drainage remedy working on the liver, kidneys and gall bladder and *Silica* was used as a deeper remedy.

22.3.93 - Much better. No pain or digging in the back. Nasty taste gone. Better mentally. All gall bladder problems totally cleared up. No remedy given.

25.5.93 - Report from patient's sister with gall bladder problem. She said patient had no further trouble and had been called by the hospital to have her gall bladder removed but she said she was perfect thanks to homœopathy and didn't need the operation. Hospital were "dumbfounded".

Case 23
Early Menopause.
9.6.94 - A woman of 34 years came having had an early menopause diagnosed. She suffered from hot flushes and had no periods. This appears to come from the effect of the contraceptive pill taken since 1982 with some breaks and last taken in January. There was a history of regular periods then periods five weeks apart. She had a termination in 1987 and 1990. She had symptoms of fluid retention in abdomen and breast and slight cramps before her periods. Her last period had been on March 15. She now suffered from perspiration, worse on her forehead and had hot flushes seven to ten times a day. In April these had been every half an hour. She felt much more tired than usual Blood tests showed that she had started the menopause and should not have any more periods.
Remedies given: *Folliculinum* descending over two days followed by *Folliculinum* 30, *Berberis* 30 and *Sepia* for five days. One week break followed by *Psorinum* descending over two days and *Hepar sulph* 30, *Kali phos* 30 and *Pulsatilla* 30 for the next five days.
25.7.94 - Had two periods two weeks apart. Hot flushes stopped. Less fluid retention otherwise periods had been normal. The tiredness went two days after she started taking the tablets. Finished the remedies three weeks ago. Remedies now given: *Tuberculinum* descending over two days followed by *Hepar sulph* 30, *Kali phos* 30 and *Pulsatilla* 30 for five days.
1.9.94 - Periods now appear normal.

ALLERGIES

A few words may be said about the treatment of allergies. It is now considered that allergies may date from a faulty eradication of foetal defence anti-bodies. This means that we are born allergic but that capacity is latent and the allergic response may be seen in later life. It may be triggered by acute diseases, by stress, traumas or a change in life's circumstances. Miasmatically allergies are tubercular and carcinogenic.We prescribe normal constitutional treatment using remedies already mentioned, e.g. *Psorinum, Hepar sulph, Rhus tox* and ensuring

CLASSICAL HOMŒOPATHY REVISITED

that *Tuberculinum* and *Carcinosin* are used. A food allergy will often improve with just this regime. Otherwise we will use in potency the substance which brings on the problem in order to reverse the effect, eradicating the production of antibodies to harmless substances.

Much of this work was pioneered by Austin White of Australia who reported over 90% success rate in young children diminishing with age to about 50% success rate in fifty year olds, continuing to decrease with age. He used the allergic substance (e.g. milk) in the 30, 200 and 1M potencies. Viz *Milk* 30 one each night for three nights; seven day gap; *Milk* 200 one each night for three nights; seven day gap; *Milk* 1M one each night for three nights. Remain off the allergic substance for a further four weeks before introducing them again gradually.

We have used both ascending and descending potencies with equal rates of success. Whilst some substances can be used together, it is probably best to use them separately and certainly not to use an organic and inorganic remedy together, (e.g. house dust and house dust mite). If at a later date there is any return of the allergy, single doses of the 5M or 10M will normally resolve the problem.

The preceding cases are not designed so much to teach a methodology but to show how the five sides of a homœopathic prescription (nosodes, dyscrasia, drainage, symptom picture and depth) may be integrated. It will be apparent however, that we use a structure of two main methodologies or a mixture of them.

We are beginning to use drainage remedies with increasing frequency as we are made more and more aware of the toxic states of our patients as a result of previous drug therapy, environmental pollution and food additives. This means that there are advantages in starting with the intensive short courses because we are able to give the indicated remedy as well as a dyscrasia and drainage remedy within the first week.

The advantage of the longer course using all remedies in descending potency is that each remedy is maximised to its full potential The disadvantage of course, is that patients will often wait over two weeks before taking the indicated remedy. This will not usually be a problem as most people will improve after taking the initial psoric and dyscrasia remedy.

APPENDIX ONE

MATERIA MEDICA

The following are a few of the remedies we use time and time again on the basis of their symptomatology, alongside the nosodes, dyscrasia, drainage and deeper acting remedies.

CARBO ANIMALIS

Contemporary materia medicas make much of the symptom picture of *Carbo animalis*, whilst our old materia medicas will put more emphasis on its deep and long action and its slow pace of action dealing with complaints that come on insidiously, develop slowly, become chronic and may be malignant.

The stony hard glands may resemble those of Belladonna, but you can never mistake one for another. Patients who are showing indications for *Belladonna* have their condition characterised by its suddenness and vitality. Where *Carbo animalis* is needed there is no vitality, everything is slowed down. Kent says that there are no rapid changes and even the inflammatory process is a passive one with the body having no tendency to repair itself.

Ulcers may slowly appear as there is a breakdown in the

constitution's ability to provide nutrients to the tissues. But there is often little or no suppuration in any condition. Suppuration is a cleansing process and the body is too weak and feeble to start this healing process.

Carbo animalis has therefore been used palliatively in cancerous and incurable cases and Kent called it a great palliative for the pains of cancer.

Carbo animalis is made from destroyed animal tissue and is therefore, one of our deepest syphilitic remedies. It is not one which we should use too soon in a case and it would be difficult to conceive using it for any acute or sub-acute condition.

Indeed it is probably the final remedy for us to use in conditions like cancers, leg ulcers, osteo-arthritis and osteoporosis. It took a long time for its provers to manifest symptoms and we should not expect to see changes too quickly from its use. After the judicious use of *Carbo animalis* we would not wish to use another remedy for some time, but rather wait to see what the body was now capable of achieving. Similarly we would not wish to repeat *Carbo animalis* for many months due to its lengthy period of action.

However, after having waited for a judicious amount of time, we will have prepared the ground for a more superficial indicated plant remedy to work more thoroughly and satisfactorily.

CAUSTICUM
Causticum is one of our deepest medicines. It contains, chemically, much *Kali phos* and because of this, according to Pritam Singh, it is perhaps our deepest drainage remedy working profoundly on the liver and kidneys. We have found some inveterate and stubborn cases (a case of acne immediately springs to mind), which seemed to refuse to improve until attention was paid to nutrition and giving *Berberis* followed by *Kali phos* followed by *Causticum* in descending potency on a daily basis.

It has 'gradually' as one of its chief characteristics. Regardless of how well it covers the symptomatology of a case it is likely to be of little use in conditions that come on quickly and are generally regarded as transient. It is a remedy for old broken down constitutions suffering from a wide variety of chronic diseases which progress slowly and where the patient is slowly deteriorating. They grow weaker. Any organ can show a decrease in function, or muscular power or paralysis. This paralysis of function can cause a shutting down of bladder, tongue (with stammering), peristaltic activity with throat and digestive problems ensuing. Paralysis can also mean stiffness and after using such indicated remedies as *Rhus tox*, deeper remedies may continue the work in rheumatism, arthritis, sciatica, etc., to produce a cure. The remedy can also encompass its opposite modality and so extreme sensitivity to pain, noise, touch, excitement or anything unusual may result.

Along with a slow deterioration of physical function there is also the anxiety, fear, melancholy and sense of hopelessness which can come on with a deterioration of the physical frame. This can progress to hysteria. Not the hysteria which comes on after an acute shock, but rather the gradual hysteria showing a breakdown of mental faculties as well as physical ones. This lead Kent to write, "*Causticum* has cured insanity, not acute manias with violent delirium, but mental aberration of the passive kind, while the brain has become tired. The constitution has been broken down with long suffering and much trouble and finally the mind is in confusion".

Almost any deep acting remedy is by definition going to be multi-miasmatic. *Causticum* is no exception. Hahnemann considered that much of the cause of psora lay in the suppression of generations of skin diseases. Kent talks of the curative action of *Causticum* where the suppression of eruptions brings our mental symptoms of exhaustion, hopelessness and despair. He also refers to the sycotic symptoms of warts and catarrh, (here its action as a drainage remedy can be very effective), as well as the syphilitic conditions of fissures and indolent ulcers.

HEPAR SULPH

We have discussed already the use of *Hepar sulph* as a dyscrasia remedy for the constitutional affects caused by mercury and other metals. Hahnemann refers to it regularly in, "Chronic Diseases" and spoke of the need to repeat it at regular intervals during treatment. In its own right it is a deep acting anti-psoric mineral remedy, but it also has, as do all mineral remedies, its anti-sycotic and anti-syphilitic side. Mercury was a general treatment for all manner of syphilitic conditions in Hahnemann's day and so an antidote to its harmful affects had obvious value. People are not all equally sensitive to the effects of mercury in amalgam fillings and so *Hepar sulph* is highly prized above other antidotes for mercury because of its keynote symptoms of sensitivity and oversensitvity. The writer remembers a case of a clairvoyant who was so oversensitive to the effects of electrical appliances that she could not even vacuum her home without unpleasant sensations. Her menstrual cycle also began to coincide with her dogs going on heat! *Hepar sulph* was given for this exceptional sensitivity, with the result that as she became more 'grounded', she began to lose some of her supersensitive clairvoyant ability.

Nash says of *Hepar sulph* that, "Its strongest characteristic is its hyper sensitiveness to touch, pain and cold air. The patient is so sensitive to pain that she faints away, even when it is slight." But we do not need to limit the things to which *Hepar sulph* is oversensitive. We are living in an allergic age. Our bodies are becoming oversensitive to chemicals and other substances and this remedy can help fortify the body against such environmental influences. Mentally too the patient can be oversensitive which can manifest in touchiness, irritability, anger, or being extremely moved by tales of misfortune. In this way *Hepar sulph* may be similar to *Nux vomica*, but deeper acting and appropriate where the constitution is more profoundly affected. Even in the digestive tract *Nux vomica* has indigestion from rich and spicy foods whilst *Hepar sulph* has a more chronic dyspepsia from the same indigestible foods which both remedies may crave.

Naturally the opposite polarity is also true and for *Hepar sulph* we also have a lack of sensitivity on the physical, mental and emotional plains. Atony of any organ is possible; that of the bowels and urinary organs being most frequently documented. It is a useful remedy in such conditions as post viral syndrome where there is a total lack of reaction.

This under functioning, of course, leads us to think of the psoric side of *Hepar sulph* and Nash says, "This is one of our strongest anti-psorics and for that reason would be thought of for all respiratory ailments for which it has such a strong affinity, especially when such ailments have followed a suppressed ...eruption on the skin."

Nash continues in his "Leaders" to explain how *Hepar sulph* is useful for the scrofulous diathesis, consumption, and is a tubercular remedy dealing with latent psora. Its sycotic side shows in the catarrh and the amelioration from damp, whilst its power over the suppurative stage of inflammations shows its ability to be anti-syphilitic in preventing deterioration and decay. *Hepar sulph* follows *Mercurius* well and is one of the best remedies after *Mercurius* either in homœopathic practice, or as an antidote to poisoning by the crude metal.

Chemically *Hepar sulph* contains *Calc carb* and may be considered to stand half way between those two great anti-psorics; *Calc carb* and *Sulphur*. Hahnemann advocated starting certain syphilitic cases with it for just those reasons mentioned above.

HYPERICUM PERFORATUM (ST JOHN'S WORT)

The action of this remedy centres on the nerves and skin. The plant has petals which when crushed exude a reddish juice and the leaves when held up to the light appear made up of little perforations. According to the 'Doctrine of Signatures' early herbalists used it as a wound remedy and this idea has been confirmed by provings and clinical trials.

It is best known as a first aid remedy and is considered for all nerve pains following shock or accident. This remedy is specially related to nerve trauma or to injuries of parts rich in nerves e.g. when finger ends have been bruised, lacerated or crushed by a hammer, or a nail has been torn off. As a result the nerves may become inflamed and there may be shooting, darting pains from the region of injury towards the body, traceable along the course of the nerve. Wounds which gape, swell up, look red and inflamed, dry, shiny on the edges, with burning, tearing and stinging pains with no tendency to heal need this remedy. Also keep it in mind when old scars get injured or torn internally with stinging, tearing, burning pains. Another useful field for the application of this remedy is spinal injuries, especially injuries of the coccyx. Here and in nerve trauma this remedy claims preference over *Arnica*.

However, chronically we have also found it successful in helping with the nerve pain from ulcers, trigeminal neuralgia and especially arthritis, sometimes in alternation with *Symphytum*.

LYCOPODIUM

Lycopodium is one of the deepest acting plant remedies with a very broad sphere of action. This makes it a good bridge remedy to some of our deeper mineral based remedies. It is produced from a moss which clings to the rocks on which it grows, making it a plant rich in many vital mineral salts.

It is not a remedy having the acute functional symptoms of *Nux vomica*, nor the broken down constitution of *Causticum* or *Carbo animalis*, but it is a remedy standing midway between the two. A driven individual needing *Nux vomica* considers that their body can go on for ever. Those needing *Causticum* know that their body has broken down. Those needing *Lycopodium* have discovered that they are not immortal, that their bodies do not contain the secret of eternal youth and with this comes the realisation that something is not functioning perfectly, or the fear that some organ or system may breakdown.

Because of its depth of action, practitioners are often warned against using *Lycopodium* as an opening remedy in high potencies as it has been known to produce acute aggravations if given too soon. It enters deeply into the life, to use the language of Kent, and almost any system or organ may be affected by it. Soft tissue, blood vessels, bones, liver, heart, joints, stomach, intestines, chest may all be acted upon by *Lycopodium*. It may be the under functioning of psora, the catarrh or growths of sycosis, or the necrosis, abscesses, spreading ulcers and emaciation of psoro-syphilis.

The rheumatic pains which may be ameliorated by motion and warmth and are accompanied by restlessness are identical to *Rhus tox* but on a deeper level.

With the worry of increasing ill health comes nervous excitement, prostration, a tired state of mind and body and unceasing anxiety that their system will break down. This leads to a lack of self-confidence and the well known characteristics of *Lycopodium* such as a growing apprehension of appearing in public. This can lead to them putting on a healthy and confident front, but the feeling is always there that something will break down and they will be found out! Feebleness is the word Kent uses to illustrate the centre of gravity of the remedy. They consider that their future looks black, they are sensitive about the fragility of their condition. Fragility is another word like feebleness covering both their physical and mental state.

We have used this remedy frequently for children with eczema with good results but never as a first remedy. Kent says, "It will throw out a greater amount of eruption at first, but this will subside finally and the child will return to health." To attempt to prevent such aggravations we will normally start our eczema cases with *Rhus tox* or *Pulsatilla* and include indicated drainage remedies before introducing the deeper *Lycopodium*.

Kent goes on to describe the catarrhal eye, ear, nose, throat and chest symptoms which make *Lycopodium* such a useful remedy. These may be symptoms that are inherited or come on after pneumonia, bronchitis or another deep seated illness. The body appears to have no tendency to repair itself. "It is especially suitable in old age and in premature old age, when a person at sixty years appears to be eighty years, broken down, feeble and tired. It is eminently suited in complaints of weakly constitutions", (Kent's "Lectures on Materia Medica").

NUX VOMICA

Boericke in his "Materia Medica" calls this remedy, "the greatest polycrest". This is because it is a medicine with a wide range of symptomatology which can be related to stress, mental strain, anxiety and worry. Pathology may be related to the digestive tract, from burping and bad breath at one end, to stomach ulcers, piles, constipation or diarrhoea at the other. There are many types of headaches as well as respiratory symptoms including coughs and asthma. The word 'spasm' is a key word of this remedy, be it a spasm of the respiratory tract affecting breathing, or a spasm of the digestive tract bringing cramps or constipation.

Nux vomica traditionally fits the picture of the typical irritable sedentary businessman (or woman) who lives on his nerves and works long hours. He is competitive and fastidious in the pursuit of excellence or promotion. He may need alcohol to unwind at the end of the day and coffee to stimulate him to action at the start of the day. Accordingly, his digestion suffers as does his sleep as he wakes too early with business on his mind

However this stereotype can severely limit our use of this remedy. Many conditions can be either caused by stress, or at least worsened by stress. An asthma problem caused by stress can be cured by *Nux vomica*, an asthma problem exacerbated by stress can be improved by *Nux vomica*, and then other deeper acting remedies must follow it to act on the predisposition. Medical reports will tell us that a legion of complaints can be stress related, which makes *Nux vomica* one of our most important and most frequently used remedies.

The following case is a typical one using *Nux vomica* and then slightly deeper remedies to follow:

Man born April 1957. X-ray showed narrowing of the large bowel. Irritable bowel syndrome started end of 1991, stress related. Loose bowel movements twice daily - watery. Flatulent, rumbling, gurgling, offensiveness which is consistently bad. Dental fillings previous year.

Prescription: Descending potencies starting at 10M then downwards through 1M, 200, 30, 18, 12, 6c taken 24 hourly, one potency each day, the remedies following on from each other in the following order:-
> *Psorinum, Hepar sulph, Nux vomica, Tuberculinum,*
> *Lycopodium.*

Six weeks later - 90% better. Bowels and general well being better immediately and improvement had been maintained. Prescription given in the same format as above with the following remedies:-
> *Psorinum, Hepar Sulph, Nux Vomica, Medorrhinum,*
> *Natrum Sulph.*

Sycotic remedies were given because of family history as well as symptoms.

The patient was heard of about a year later when he visited the clinic for a massage and all symptoms had remained well.

PULSATILLA (MEADOW ANEMONE)
When we consider conditions which are linked with the female hormonal system, we will often think of the dyscrasia remedy *Folliculinum*. However the two main remedies to use accordingly to their symptomatology are *Sepia* and *Pulsatilla*. One is an animal derivative, the other from a plant and they are remedies which complement each other, following on and completing what the other remedy has started.

Pulsatilla affects especially the mucous membranes, respiratory system and the female sex hormones. Pre-eminently, though not exclusively, it is a remedy for women and children, prescribed very much on its mental and emotional symptoms. As a hormonal remedy it is comparable with *Sepia* but the emotional picture is entirely different.

Pulsatilla can be a very dependent person with mildness, tearfulness and indecisiveness. There is a need for consolation and company, to such a degree that patients may be so manipulative as to stop her parents or friends from leaving her even temporarily. There can also be marked jealousy if someone else is getting the attention she feels she ought to have. Usually however, they are gentle people with changeable moods, easily upset and with a degree of self-pity. The word 'clingy' is often used by their parents to describe a *Pulsatilla* child, and here, whether they are suffering from an infectious disease, a chest infection of earache, *Pulsatilla* is likely to help. It is an important rheumatic remedy with characteristic shifting, changing, wandering pains. There is a changeability of physical symptoms, as well as of their emotional nature. There are many circulatory disorders including chilblains and varicose veins (also *Hamamelis*). There can be heartburn and a nasty bitter taste in the mouth and chronic indigestion with spasm in the stomach and abdominal region. A tendency to colitis and alternating constipation and diarrhoea is common. *Pulsatilla* is an antidote to the overeating of too fatty foods. It is good in cases of catarrh, either of the respiratory system or the alimentary tract. Discharges are usually bland and thick and yellow or greenish yellow. Many menstrual disorders will respond to *Pulsatilla*. The periods are generally irregular, delayed and scanty. Many complaints of puberty and pregnancy as well as some cases of pre-menstrual tension and menopause will call for this remedy. Always remember however, the need to match the emotional symptoms.

Pulsatilla should not be forgotten for men, and a look at the materia medica shows that many problems of the testicles will respond to it. It is called for in patients who are anaemic or who have taken too many iron tonics even years before. Finally *Pulsatilla* is an important skin remedy and may be tried for many cases of dry eczema, unlike the oozing of *Rhus tox*.

RADIUM BROMIDE

Radium as a homœopathic remedy was discovered by the son and daughter-in-law of a well known Parisian homœopath. It was named because of its great radiating power and it is now a remedy in everyday practice. It is a useful remedy due to its wide range of action, depth of action and because of its use as a dyscrasia remedy.

Clarke in his booklet, *"Radium* as an Internal Remedy" wrote, "The tremendous energy thrown out by *Radium* will naturally suggest to the homœopath a centrifugal action in an antipsoric effect - in throwing central diseases out upon the skin.". He goes on to cite many cured skin cases ranging from various forms to eczema to psoriasis, pruritis, acne and acne rosacea.

The first proving was done with the crude element by M. Curie who said, "If there is one thing I know about Radium, it is that it will burn". He put a small amount of the salt in an india rubber capsule and left it attached to his arm for ten hours. This turned into an ulcer which took four months to heal. On another occasion he attached it for half an hour and an ulcer appeared after two weeks which took two further weeks to heal, and on a third occasion he attempted the experiment for just eight minutes - two months later there was soreness and inflammation in that area.

We see here the deep syphilitic nature of the remedy which is able to produce and cure ulcerous conditions, as well as the slow pace of action of the remedy. Inflammations of an acute nature are best dealt with by such as *Belladonna*, leaving *Radium bromide* from the more intractable long standing conditions.

The remedy's success with the sycotic conditions of catarrh and warts are well documented. Dr. Dieffenbach stated, "catarrhal or intestinal nephritis, with rheumatic symptoms corresponding to the provings, has apparently been beneficial". He then went on to draw attention to its use for symptoms of the respiratory tract, especially the persistent cough which occurred late in the provings and he spoke of using *Radium bromide* in tuberculosis, whooping cough, bronchitis and pneumonia.

In addition to treating the Tubercular miasm, *Radium* has been used with some success in treating cancer. Indeed Clarke devotes a whole chapter to the use of the potentised material in cancer and the cancerous diathesis. No miasm is not fully covered by this remedy.

Pritam Singh further researched this remedy in its place in the periodic table of elements. At the bottom of the group which includes barium, calcium and magnesium, he considered it to be an excellent remedy when the system has been overloaded by one of these substances. As well, of course, in its action of antidoting the effects of too many X-rays.

In this connection we use *Radium bromide* for many digestive ailments. Our patients may have purchased many proprietary magnesium based ant-acids with limited success for an over active digestive system, they were then sent by the doctor for a barium meal or barium enema and subjected to a course of X-rays. In cases such as these, *Radium bromide* may be a useful remedy given first to deal with antidoting the effect of the crude chemicals and then preparing the way for our anti-psoric and indicated remedies to work more fully.

The ingestion of crude calcium is yet another reason to use *Radium bromide*. Crude calcium can lead to kidney stones and other calcium deposits. A look at the contents of tins and bottles on supermarket shelves show a large number to have calcium added, including many forms of baby milk and baby foods. Often this is in quite an indigestible form and cases of infantile eczema can be cleared with *Radium brom* alone; though most will benefit from *Psorinum*, drainage remedies and individual remedies such as *Pulsatilla* or *Rhus tox*.

Guernsey's "Materia Medica" expounds in a few other areas. He says that it is well known that massive doses of radium produce atheroma and that many symptoms would point to its use in arterio-sclerosis. He states that all provers showed lowered blood pressure and that the use of the remedy has often been clinically verified in the treatment of high blood pressure whether of functional origin or due to organic disease. His comments at the increased elimination of solids through the urinary tract show it to be a valuable drainage remedy. He goes on to state, "Enuresis has been cured and many cases of diabetes are reported as cured".

The lassitude, tiredness and depression are frequently commented upon. An eminent homœopath used *Radium bromide* to cure many cases of post viral syndrome. He is practising in Wales where many animals had been slaughtered due to nuclear fallout from the ill fated reactor at Chernobyl, which points to a likely link between radiation and the disease.

Whilst anaemia is in part nutritional, marked changes in this condition have been seen in subjects taking *Radium bromide*. Provers have also seen an increase or decrease in erythrocytes as the action of *Radium bromide* is seen on the blood. Dr. Dieffenbach comments, "The absolute scientific fact which stands out clearly in the provings, and which can unquestionably be attributed to the drug, is the marked increase of the polymorphuclear neutrophiles. These so called policemen of the blood corpuscles are the ones which attack the invading bacteria and destroy them and the administration of *Radium bromide* appears to have distinctly stimulated the organism in the elaboration and increase of these protection organisms."

Guernsey concludes his essay by telling us that *Radium bromide* does not interfere with the action of other indicated remedies but rather enhances them and advocates the use of this element as an intercurrent remedy.

RHUS TOX

This is one of our most well-known remedies in the materia medica. Its symptomatolgy equates to most conditions of rheumatism and rheumatoid arthritis, i.e. the muscle pains are worse cold/damp, better for heat, hot baths and massage, much worse on first movement and better for continual motion unless they over exert themselves.

However so often practitioners use *Rhus tox* based solely on the symptom picture and so often they are disappointed with the results. A well known homœopathic company markets rheumatism tablets which are simply *Rhus tox* in the 6th potency. Some patients get relief with these, but again many do not. I hear practitioners say that they do not like treating rheumatism because they almost never get good results.

At our clinic we continually see improvements and cures with rheumatism. We may use nutrition as well but homœopathically we use *Rhus tox* and we make it work. Many practitioners fail to make it work because they do not understand that it is made from the tincture of the fresh leaves and is therefore, not a particularly deep acting remedy, despite the fact that rheumatoid arthritis is usually a very deep seated condition. Remedies like

Appendix I

Lycopodium and *Tuberculinum* have similar symptomatology and will help *Rhus tox* to work on a more profound level.

As rheumatic complaints are caused by a toxic blood stream, the importance of using drainage remedies with such conditions cannot be over emphasised.

Rhus tox is made from a variety of poison ivy, which is a plant responsible for causing some of the most allergic reactions known that can affect the skin and respiratory tract. People responsible for clearing patches of the plant have suffered from all manner of itching skin conditions, respiratory conditions and tiredness.

Allen comments on the periodicity of its symptomatolgy in the provings and says that the toxic effects of the crude plant seem ineradicable without anti-psoric treatment. He had a case where a patient had an annual return of her symptoms after being poisoned with poison ivy which was only cured by monthly does of *Tuberculinum.*

The eye symptoms of *Rhus tox* are worthy of note because there are few eye conditions which can be successfully treated homœopathically, which will not respond to *Rhus tox, Ruta* or *Pulsatilla.*

Rhus tox is one of the main remedies which we use for a myriad of different kinds of allergic conditions; whatever the cause, along with *Psorinum, Tuberculinum* and other indicated remedies to make it work on a more profound level. Sometimes an apparently indicated eczema or hay fever remedy may yield disappointing results. Further questioning of the patient will reveal that in his or her parents, grandparents and relations is the *Rhus tox* symptom complex of the asthma, eczema, hay fever, allergic rashes, etc. Here *Rhus tox* will cover the whole picture and bring encouraging results. As 'stress' is a keynote for *Nux vomica* so 'allergy' is a keynote word for *Rhus tox.*

The following case illustrates how *Rhus tox* can be used in conjunction with other remedies to treat babies and very young children.

27.2.92 - Baby boy born May 1990. Eczema and asthma in family background.

Itchy eczema. Warm bath ameliorates. Started as a dribble rash in previous year. Blisters at first. Immunisation two months prior to onset. Frequent colds.

Prescription: Remedies given 24 hourly in descending potencies, CM or 10M downwards, one potency a day through 1M, 200, 30, 18, 12 and 6c:-

Psorinum, Hepar sulph, Rhus tox, Tuberculinum.

1.4.92 - Much improved. Still dry but redness gone. Chest much better than arms, (Hering's Law of Cure). Aggressive and ratty at first and slight runny nose at beginning of remedies. Urinating more. Sleeping less. (This shows that the body's processes of elimination have been stimulated). After one week's break the following was given in the same way as above:-

Psorinum, Hepar sulph, Rhus tox, Tuberculinum

Followed by *Hepar sulph* 30 in the morning and *Rhus tox* 30 in the evening.

8.6.92 - Eczema clear on holiday. Red and sore on return, then cleared up. Better now than at any time since treatment started. Remedies were again given in the same descending way as follows:

Psorinum, Hepar Sulph, Rhus Tox, Medorrhinum. Lycopodium.

The next appointment was cancelled as the boy was totally well.

SANICULA AND THE AQUA REMEDIES

Clarke says, "we have in *Sanicula* one of the best proved remedies of the materia medica and an antipsoric of wide range".

Generally, however, this remedy is little known. The reason is that its symptom picture is so wide and diverse that it is difficult to speak of a specific *Sanicula* symptomatolgy. This is because *Sanicula*, made from mineral water from Illinois, is polypharmacy in a single remedy. *Sanicula aqua* is rich in Sodium chloride , Calc. mur., Mag. mur., Calc. bicarb., Calc sulph., Kali.sulph., Nat.bicarb., Nat.brom., Ferrum bicarb., Natrum iod., Silica and Alumina with traces of Lithium bicarb., Nat.phos. and Borax. Its provings therefore mimic all of these remedies. As these salts are contained in diluted form it is not one of our deepest remedies, but can extend the action of many of our plant remedies helping them to work more profoundly.

In a recent case a practitioner was lead to prescribe *Sanicula* because of a child's craving for bottled water, she was not assimilating the mineral salts well from her food. Indeed one word to give distinctiveness to the provings of the mineral waters would be 'malassimilation'. Dr Schussler's theory of the biochemic mineral salts was that health depends on the assimilation of the organic and inorganic and that giving certain mineral salts in a readily assimilable form could help to supercede the body's own salt solution. He considered that much of disease was caused by a poor assimilation of certain inorganic salts. Whilst this must, to some degree remain as disputed theory, there are many symptoms of *Sanicula* linked with the keynote of malassimilation; the failure to thrive or put on weight, delayed development, the emaciation despite a large appetite, marasmus, large swollen abdomen, coeliac disease, etc.

Obviously we see here the under functioning of psora, but like any mineral remedy, we shall see numerous characteristics of the other miasms. And so we find as examples, the marked sycotic catarrh and discharges with a fishy odour which remind us of *Medorrhinum* and the mouth ulcers reminding us of *Mercurius* and the syphilitic remedies.

Wiersbaden comes from the water of a spring in Prussia containing a similar richness of minerals and salts to *Sanicula*: Potassium, Sodium, Lithium, Ammonium, Magnesium, Iron, Manganese, Silica, Strontium and Copper. Because of this it can be used almost interchangeably with Sanicula. It has not had such a thorough proving and many homœopaths know about it for its symptom of hair loss, but here we see that the condition of the hair is a good indication of the failure of the body to absorb important nutrients.

Skookum chuck is a Native American name for what the Indians consider to be a lake of strong medicinal properties. It was known for its cure of psoric skin diseases by those who bathed in it and drank the water, as well as helping many multi-miasmatic conditions like hay fever where the psora is uppermost.

SEPIA (INK OF CUTTLEFISH)
Although the first known proving of *Sepia* was by a man who continually licked the tip of his brush which had previously been dipped into sepia ink, this is predominantly a female remedy. A study of its provings will show that it includes many

symptoms common to both the menopause with its hot flushes, as well as many other physical and mental discomforts found at certain times of the menstrual cycle. There is weakness of the pelvic organs with irregular periods and great pressure and bearing down sensations. Headaches, weakness, tiredness and a loss of libido are common concomitant symptoms. *Sepia* is also a major remedy for leucorrhoea and thrush.

Sepia is a common remedy for the nausea of pregnancy (also *Pulsatilla* and *Nux vomica*), with an empty sinking feeling and nausea at the thought and smell of food. There may be inactivity of the rectum and protruding piles. *Sepia* is commonly used in cystitis and bladder problems (also *Thuja* and *Medorrhinum*). With *Sepia* there may be frequent urination, and the urine can be very offensive. There can be enuresis of children during the first sleep (also *Petroleum*).

Sepia has many skin symptoms often linked to the hormonal cycle. In psoriasis, if there are red spots before the scales and especially brown liver spots on the abdomen and chest think of *Sepia*. It will also cover many cases of female acne. In cases of prolapsed organs, depending on the degree of pathology we will first give *Nux vomica* and then *Sepia*.

With *Sepia* there is stasis, a lack of certain feminine qualities, as if that which makes them womanly has not developed or has been worn down by the ravages of life. They may feel that they become a doormat for their family to whom they develop an indifference, and they become irritable if any pressure is put upon them. They feel a need for space and to get away from all the pressures of life. There is no enjoyment of life and they can become melancholy, wallow in self-pity and be very tearful, worse company and consolation (the opposite of *Pulsatilla*). Consider *Sepia* in cases of sterility where other symptoms agree. The circulation is poor and they may often catch colds. Their chilliness makes this a useful remedy in Raynaud's Syndrome. *Sepia* is a liver remedy and may often feel better from violent exercise when the liver is shaken about.

Case of Mrs C, who was born in November 1973. Her grandmother, mother and twin sisters all suffered from pre-menstrual tension and bad periods. Before her period she complained of nausea, tiredness, worry, panic, touchiness and knew that she became irrational; like a Jeckell and Hyde character. She was fine before going on the pill. She wanted bread and 'stodge' before her periods and complained of chest palpitations when the period arrived. She had received many mercury fillings during her life. Her prescription was:-

Day 1	*Psorinum* 10M, 1M, 200
Day 2	*Psorinum* 30, 12, 6
Day 3 - 7	*Hepar sulph* 30 - morning
	Berberis 30 - afternoon
	Sepia 30 - evening
Days 8 - 14	Nil
Day 15	*Folliculinum* 10M, 1M, 200
Day 16	*Folliculinum* 30, 12, 6
Day 17 - 21	*Folliculinum* 30 - morning
	Berberis 30 - afternoon
	Sepia 30 - evening

A month later, "A lot better". She declared herself calmer with less PMT, and was less depressed. The period and pains were better. She experienced no palpitations and was eating more normally before the period. She was given, in descending potencies, on a daily basis:-

Psorinum, Hepar sulph, Sepia and then *Tuberculinum.*

Six weeks later she considered herself fine, without problems. She had got over a cold quicker than normal and was in no need of further treatment.

SPONGIA TOSTA

Spongia is made from a very primitive sea animal which is heated, or toasted, before being made into a remedy. It has been found that where heat is used in the manufacture of a remedy we have a substance working on a deeper level. Other such remedies being *Carbo animalis, Carbo veg., Causticum* and *Phosphorus.* Hahnemann found that a proving of smelted aluminium produced quite different symptoms to that of normal aluminium. Today people are experimenting in producing deeper acting remedies made from the ash of a whole plant, whilst previously just part of the plant may have been triturated and succussed in the normal way.

Spongia is, therefore, one of our deeper remedies. As it is a creature of the sea, soaking up the elements of sea water, it is rich in iodine as well as containing *Bromine, Calc. phos., Calc.*

carb., Potassium iod., Aluminium, Sulphur, Silica, Sodium chloride.
There is also spongin; a fibrous keratin-like material found only in natural sponges.

Parallels may be drawn between this remedy and those produced from mineral waters, which we have just discussed, but with the cells of the sponge being fed by sea water the iodine content is much larger (1.5 - 14%), which is liberated by the roasting process.

Because of what it contains, *Spongia* is a remedy of use in a wide variety of conditions. Its effects on respiration, with the patient feeling as if they were breathing through a sponge, croupy coughs, croup, heart valvular complaints, angina, testicle problems, skin and bone problems are all widely documented. However, whilst there are many similar polycrests for some conditions, *Spongia* is invaluable for many afflictions of the thyroid glands.

Goitre is marked, being related to the presence of bromine and iodine which the sponge contains. Indeed goitre used to be most common in areas furthest from the sea as the food was less rich in iodine. *Spongia* covers many of the symptoms of thyroid imbalance, including: neck, gland and eye symptoms as well as the restlessness or weariness, the temperature reactions and weight loss or gain.

Pritam Singh considered constitutional thyroid problems to be tubercular in origin and certainly most of our classical homœopaths have referred to the tubercular nature of *Spongia*. This in itself shows it to have a depth of action. Many of its symptoms are seen as being classically tubercular such as its, "changeability, stubbornness, disorientatation, lack of tolerance, aggravation at night, respiratory disease, dryness of body and cough and glandular enlargement and induration". Also its ability to deal with caries of the bone, points to its tubercular/syphilitic nature. (Jo Evans, "Spongia tosta - A Study of its Signatures", The Homœopath No 611996).

SYMPHYTUM OFFICINALE (COMFREY, KNITBONE)

Think of this remedy for bruised periosteum (also *Ruta*) and fractured bones, also for injuries of the eye ball and the surrounding bone (orbital periosteum). In eye injuries there is hardly any remedy to excell this, it will prevent traumatic cataract and the ensuing blindness. In injuries of parts where the bone is near the skin e.g. the cheeks and the face, or the shin. It hastens the formation of the callus and thus expedites the union of fractured bones. Because of its affinity with bone material and ability to encourage bone formation it is used in chronic conditions such as osetoporosis and osteo-arthritis as a first indicated remedy, followed with deeper acting mineral remedies such as *Calc phos, Silica* and *Carbo animalis.*

THUJA OCCIDENTALIS (YELLOW CEDAR)

The primary areas of action of *Thuja* are the nervous system, the mucous membranes (those membranes of the genito-urinary tract in particular) and the lymphatic system. This is another very important polycrest remedy and, as previously discussed will go a long way towards clearing the dyscrasia of vaccination and also that left by gonorrhoea. It is also a good remedy for non-malignant and warty growths. Its use is invaluable for the treatment of the sycotic miasm, being deeper acting than *Medorrhinum,* and can be used in descending potencies to prepare the way for a remedy based on symptomatology.

This remedy, dealing as it does with over-production in the system will be thought of in many cases of catarrh and sinus problems (along with *Hepar sulph*). It is also a fundamental remedy for genito-urinary tract and prostrate problems. Symptoms include: inflammation of the lymph glands, swelling in the groin and perspiration of an unpleasant nature. It is an important rheumatic remedy. Notable sensations include: hot burning sensations alternating with cold, pins and needles in the extremities and twitching and cramping of the muscles.

On the emotional front there can be depression. They may appear sensitive and temperamental in company as though they have something to hide, they often dislike company and can be quarrelsome with fixed ideas.

Thuja precedes *Tuberculinum* well and will often be helped by the addition of *Tuberculinum* where it is indicated.

Much of conventional homœopathy is based solely on discovering the symptom picture. However, we have found many cases ranging from catarrh to urinary problems which have totally cleared up using the nosodes of *Psorinum* and *Tuberculinum* and the dyscrasia remedies of *Hepar sulph* and *Thuja*. Once remedies have been given to assist the body in shedding its toxic load the person's vital energy can be stimulated to work curatively to bring about healing without any further help from potentised remedies.

APPENDIX TWO

THERAPEUTICS

Over the years we have found the following aide memoire helpful. We do not adhere to it in any slavish way, but we give below remedies which have stood us in good stead if no other remedies are obviously indicated. The core therapeutics listed below does not take into account the depth of action of remedies and should be read alongside Chapter 5.

ACNE   *Calc carb* or *Hepar sulph, Tuberculinum*
ABSCESS   *Hepar sulph, Zinc phos, Silica*
ADDISON'S DISEASE   *Gelsemium* (fast and short acting) or
    Rhus tox
ALCOHOL CRAVING   *Syphillinum, Nux vomica.*
ANKYLOSING SPONDILITIS   *Symphytum*
ALLERGIES   *Rhus tox, Zinc phos.*
ASTHMA   *Calc carb* or *Hepar sulph. Arsenicum album* if no
    dyscrasia or mercury fillings and few symptoms.
    Otherwise *Rhus tox.* Occasionally *Pulsatilla, Sepia*
    or other indicated remedy. *Baptisia* for acute
    attack. Bronchial catarrhal asthma - *Sabal serrulata.*

ATHEROMA *Radium bromide*
BED WETTING   *Hepar sulph* or *Calc carb* with *Petroleum,*
          Tuberculinum, and *Syphillinum*
BLOOD DISORDERS   *Ferrum phos*
BOILS   *Hepar sulph*
BURNS   *Psorinum, Hepar sulph, Cantharis.* Pour on
          Cantharis 30 diluted. *Carbo animalis.* Dyscrasia
          from old burns *Carbo animalis.*
CANDIDA   *Psorinum, Tuberculinum, Hepar sulph, Penicillinum*
CAR SICKNESS   *Petroleum, Cocculus*
CARTILAGE   *Ruta* (Deep problems that *Rhus tox* does not reach)
CATARRH *Pulsatilla* if symptoms agree. *Thuja.* (*Thuja* and
          Pulsatilla may antidote each other so should not
          be given at the same time).
CHANGING SYMPTOMS   *Tuberculinum*
CHEST INFECTION   *Carbo animalis* if severe
CHILDREN CONSTITUTIONALLY - *Calc phos* up to 18
          (Mental at expense of physical and vice versa).
CHILDREN'S DISEASES*Psorinum, Tuberculinum*
CHOLESTEROL *Zinc phos*
CHRON'S DISEASE   *Lycopodium* followed by *Podophyllum*
          and *Silica*
COLOUR BLINDNESS   *Sabal serrulata* and *Digitalis*
CONSTIPATION Acute - *Aconite.* Chronic - *Opium, Nux vomica*
COUGH   Children - *Calc phos.* Loose - *Ant tart, Psorinum,*
          Tuberculinum
CRACKED SKIN *Hepar sulph, Petroleum*
CYSTITIS   Acute - *Medorrhinum* and *Cantharis*
          Chronic - *Sepia, Thuja, Natrum sulph*
CYSTS   *Radium bromide*
DIARRHOEA *Nux vomica* followed by *Lycopodium* and
          Podophyllum
DIETING   Comfort eating - *Lycopodium, Pulsatilla.*
DIGESTIVE   *Nux vomica, Lycopodium, Podophyllum.*
DROPSY   *Rhus tox, Apis.*
DRUG DYSCRASIA   May be *Nux vomica.* Tranquillisers -
          Zinc phos. Steroids - *Kali phos.* Sodium Based
          Drugs - *Natrum mur.*
DRUGS   Coming off - include *Avena sativa* tincture.
          Also consider drug in potency.

DUODENAL ULCERS   *Podophyllum*
ECZEMA   *Calc carb* (or *Hepar sulph* if amalgum dyscrasia)
            and *Rhus tox*. Dry- *Pulsatilla*. Include *Berberis* to
            help kidneys eliminate. Painful - *Hypericum*.
EYES   Often *Ruta*. *Rhus tox* may help.
ENDOMETRIOSIS   *Sepia* or *Pulsatilla* with *Thuja*;
            Medorrhinum
FACIAL HAIR IN WOMEN   *Sabal serrulata, Folliculinum*.
FIBROIDS   *Thuja, Phytolacca, Medorrhinum*.
GALLSTONES   *Radium bromide, Lycopodium, Nux vomica*.
GLUE EAR   *Psorinum, Tuberculinum, Pulsatilla, Rhus tox*.
GOUT   *Ledum* followed by *Rhus tox* and *Tuberculinum*.
            Arnica in acute and later stages.
HAEMORRHAGE   *Tuberculinum*. *Phosphorus* speeds
            healing of wounds and ulcers.
HAIR LOSS   *Wiersbaden*.
HAY FEVER   *Rhus tox, Psorinum, Tuberculinum*.
HEART COMPLAINTS   *Crataegus, Digitalis*.
HEAD LICE   *Psorinum* and *Tuberculinum* remove tendency.
HERPES   Nose and lips - *Natrum mur*. Face - *Rhus tox*.
            Bottom lip/chin - *Medorrhinum, Sepia*.
HORMONAL IMBALANCE   *Sepia, Pulsatilla, Thuja, Ruta*
HYDROCEPHALUS   *Podophyllum*
HIGH BLOOD PRESSURE   *Radium bromide, Psorinum*
HYPOGLYCAEMIC   *Phosphoric acid, Lycopodium, Zinc phos*
IMMUNE SYSTEM   Poor - *Hepar sulph* both for over sensi-
            tive and under sensitive.
INSOMNIA   *Piscidia* tincture - 5 drops in warm water in
            evening. Also *Valerian* and *Passiflora* tincture.
INFERTILITY *Folliculinum, Pulsatilla, Sepia, Zinc phos,*
            Natrum mur
KIDNEYS   *Berberis, Sarsaparilla*.
KIDNEY STONES   *Nux vomica, Lycopodium, Calc carb,*
            Berberis, Benzoic acid. Wounds from stones -
            Phosphorus. *Radium bromide* removes calcium.
LEUCORRHOEA *Sepia*
M.E.   *Rhus tox* for pains, stiffness, weakness,
            hopelessness.
            Insulin lifts tiredness and low blood sugar level.
            Sarcolactic acid, Phosphoric acid, Lycopodium, Zinc.

MEMORY LOSS *Cocculus*

MENIERES *China, China sulph, Psorinum, Hepar sulph.*

MENOPAUSE *Sepia, Pulsatilla, Folliculinum.*

MENSTRUAL *Sepia, Pulsatilla, Phytolacca, Ruta. Nux vomica* first
if cramping pains. *Mag sulph* for short cycles.
Carbo veg is deeper remedy. *Radium bromide*
increases red blood cells.

MORNING SICKNESS *Sepia, Nux vomica, Pulsatilla. Phosphorus*
or *Phosphoric acid* if accompanied by fainting.

M.S. *Psorinum/Hepar sulph/Rhus tox/Tuberculinum* in
first prescription. Use *Syphillinum* as a nosode in
second prescription. Also *Phosphoric acid,
Causticum, Bryonia, Cocculus.*

NIGHT TERRORS *Calc carb, Zinc phos*

OEDEMA *Rhus tox, Natrum mur, Apis.*

OSTEOARTHRITIS *Symphytum, Ledum. Lycopodium*
deeper acting.

OSTEOPOROSIS *Calc phos, Symphytum* with *Hepar sulph. Arnica*
for soft bones before age 45.

PAIN From erosion of skin or bone *Radium bromide*
then alternate*Hypericum* and *Symphytum.*

PARKINSONS *Psorinum, Hepar sulph* stimulates nerve reaction.

PILL - CONTRACEPTIVE Periods stopped - *Folliculinum,
Sepia, Cantharis*

PLEURISY *Carbo animalis*

PREGNANCY One month before birth use *Pulsatilla* 200 single
dose, followed by *Pulsatilla* 30 one a day for 7
days. Repeat in the week following birth after
Arnica This helps prevent post natal depression,
bleeding, complications, malposition, and helps
discharge of placenta. Also helps restore shape
and skin tone.
Caulophyllum 30 hourly once contractions start
until birth.
After delivery *Arnica* 30 every 10 minutes as
necessary.
Tender breasts - *Arnica.*
Radium bromide antidotes magnesium in epidu-
rals, use especially in post natal depression after
epidural.

PROLAPSE   *Nux vomica* before *Sepia*.
PSORIASIS   *Tuberculinum*. Vesicles before scales - *Rhus tox*.
Red spots before scales, especially in women,
Sepia. Also *Pulsatilla*.
PROSTATE   *Thuja, Sabal serrulata*.
PUS   Usually syphilitic. Tubercular if white watery
serum. If worse damp - Syco-syphilitic.
RAYNAUD'S SYMDROME   *Radium bromide*.
RADIATION   *Radium bromide*. *X-ray* if good vitality as this is
very deep acting.
RHEUMATISM   *Rhus tox*. *Bryonia* may follow. *Pulsatilla* for
shifting wandering, changing pains. *Cocculus* for
aches and pains below the hip area.
SINUSITIS   *Psorinum, Hepar sulph, Thuja*.
STIFFNESS/CALCIFICATION   *Radium bromide*.
SYNOVITIS   *Pulsatilla, Ledum*.
SPERM COUNT LOW *Sabal serrulata, Folliculinum*.
STERILITY   *Sepia* or *Pulsatilla* on mental symptoms then
Cantharis, Sabal serrulata, Folliculinum,
Lycopodium, Thuja, Tuberculinum.
SCAR TISSUE *Thiosinaminum*
STOMACH ULCERS   *Podophyllum, Carbo animalis*
SHINGLES   *Psorinum, Rhus tox, Tuberculinum*.
SICKLE CELL ANAEMIA   *Rhus tox, Ferrum phos* and
Syphillinum
THRUSH   *Sepia, Pulsatilla*.
THYROID   *Tuberculinum, Thyroidinum*.
TEETHING   *Calc phos*.
TRIGIUM   Growths on eye - *Argentum nit*.
TESTICLE PROBLEMS   Often *Pulsatilla*. *Spongia, Thuja, Clematis*.
ULCERS   Releasing watery serum - *Tuberculinum*. If hard-
ened edge - *Thuja*.
ULCERS - LEG   *Psorinum/Hepar sulph/Tuberculinum*. Next
prescription use *Syphillinum* as nosode. Oozing -
Rhus tox.
Consider *Phosphorus, Carbo animalis*.
VARICOSE VEINS   Women - *Pulsatilla*. *Hamamelis*.
VITILIGO   *Tuberculinum, Ars sulph flav, Carbo animalis*.
In white people consider *Penicillinum* as can be
caused by anti-biotics.

Much of the above comes originally from the research of Pritam Singh. We are not stating that the above remedies will cure the indicated conditions. What is curable depends on the extent of the pathology and the general health and vitality of the patient. All we are saying is that as far as homœopathic remedies are capable of helping patients with these conditions, then we are confident of the above remedies ability to do so.

APPENDIX THREE

POTENCY - PRACTICAL APPLICATION

The potency or strength of homœopathic potencies has always been a difficult subject. How do we find the optimum or right strength for our patient?

As potency increases so does the duration and depth of action, but the breadth of action may be lost. A high potency can obliterate the centre of the disease while a low potency may not have enough power to complete the cure. A fact that is so often overlooked is that different potencies produced different symptomatolgy when provings took place. A read of Allen's, "Keynotes" or Kent's, "Materia Medica" will often show the potency in brackets after the symptom. This points to the fact that this symptom was produced by a certain potency. To maximise the potential of a remedy, therefore, we need to give it with its complement of the full range of potencies. We commonly use the 10M, 1M, 200C, 30C, 12C and 6C potencies. Occasionally we will also use the CM potency, especially when using the nosodes which dig deeply into the inherited background.

If we are using a range of potencies on a daily basis or less frequently, we will restrict our use of the higher potencies under certain circumstances. For example we will normally start with 1M, 200 or even lower where any of the following conditions occur:-

1. The patient has a medical history of a potentially very serious or even fatal condition.
2. The patient is over 60 years of age.
3. The patient has a poor vitality and recovers very slowly from acute and chronic problems.
4. The pulse is irregular (unless medical investigations have shown that there is no underlying problem).

The more the patient shows combinations of the above, the lower the potency with which we will commence treatment. As the patient's health improves, so they will gradually be able to cope with higher potencies. However should a high potency be followed by any form of aggravation this will be curtailed by immediately giving a lower potency.

From this we learn an important principle; that there is a balance or ratio to be taken into account. One factor is the size of the potency, and on the other side of the equation, we have the length of time that it is allowed to act before a lower potency is given. It may, therefore, be perfectly in order for us to use a 10M potency for someone with a rather feeble vitality, so long as a 1M is given an hour later and a 200C an hour after that.

In practice we have two main ways of administering remedies for chronic conditions. The method we usually start with, commonly referred to as a 'Mini Programme', is to give the initial remedy - often *Psorinum* - descending down over two days; that is one dose each of 10M, 1M and 200 at hourly intervals on the first day followed by one dose each of 30C, 12C and 6C potencies at hourly intervals on the second day. As an example, we would give someone one dose of *Psorinum* 10M at 6pm, *Psorinum* 1M at 7pm and *Psorinum* 200C at 8pm on day 1. The following day, they would take *Psorinum* 30C at 6pm, *Psorinum* 12C at 7pm and *Psorinum* 6C at 8pm. We then follow up on the next five days with a dyscrasia remedy e.g. *Hepar sulph* 30C each morning, the indicated remedy in a 30C potency in the middle of each day and an organ support remedy e.g. *Berberis* 30C each evening.

Two to four weeks later, depending on the case we will follow up with a similar programme but using slightly deeper acting remedies. For instance *Tuberculinum* may be descended from 10m down to 6C over the first two days followed on the next five days by a dyscrasia remedy, the same or a related indicated remedy and a deeper organ remedy such a *Kali phos*, all again in the 30C potency.

Considerable improvement will have occurred by this time and we follow up with monthly mini programmes of deeper and deeper remedies and all the indicated nosodes.

The second method we use in chronic conditions is commonly referred to as the 'Maxi Programme'. Here we descend down through the remedies on a daily basis giving one dose of one potency each day. We would generally start with a psoric remedy, for instance one dose of *Psorinum* 10M on day one, 1M on day two, 200C on day three and so on down to 6C. We would then proceed to descend down through a dyscrasia remedy in the same way with one potency each day, followed by an indicated remedy, generally a plant remedy, again descended on a daily basis. We would then address a miasmatic layer, generally using *Tuberculinum* descended daily again in the same way and so on down through the deeper remedies. See Chapter 5, "Sounding the Depths".

We would normally start off with the 'Mini Plans' building the patient up to take higher potencies and deeper acting remedies before commencing onto a Maxi Plan. This means that by starting with a Mini Plan, not only are we normally giving the indicated remedy along with dyscrasia and drainage remedies by the third day, but we can also given our opening remedy (e.g. *Psorinum*) in high strengths but at short intervals to allow it to have its full breadth of effect. Later on as we repeat it on a daily basis in the Maxi Plan we shall see it having its full depth of effect as well. In this case the patient has already been built up, so the higher potencies can work in the system for a longer period.

We see very few aggravations even in skin conditions using these methods. Pritam Singh developed the Maxi Plans first and brought in the Mini programmes as a gentler option. Originally some patients found the high potencies of the dyscrasia remedies and the nosodes difficult to handle in the

Maxi Plans, but by using the Mini Plans first the patient is bought to a point where they are able to handle high potencies without aggravation.

Treating this way gives us great flexibility. Within a few days of starting treatment we are using indicated remedies which make the patient feel better, but at the same time letting other remedies do the donkey work of cleansing and clearing the body as well as addressing the miasmatic layer. A variety of dyscrasia remedies can be used in the Mini Plans, *Hepar sulph* probably has the widest range of action, but other remedies may be used such as *Thuja* for vaccinations, or *DPT*, *Radium bromide*, *Candida*, or *Influenzinum* depending on the case. In the same way different organ support remedies may be included in the Mini Plan; *Berberis* is important for its support of the liver and kidneys and thereby helps the initial detoxification triggered by the dyscrasia remedies. But other organ remedies can be used, even bowel nosodes to help elimination through the digestive tract if this appears to be unbalanced, this is often helpful in allergy related conditions.

As Hahanemann wrote, "The highest ideal of therapy is to restore health rapidly, gently, permanently; to remove and destroy the whole disease in the shortest, surest, least harmful way, according to clearly comprehensible principles."

APPENDIX FOUR

EXAMPLE OF PRESCRIPTION STRATEGY FOR DEALING WITH CHRONIC DISEASE

If in doubt when dealing with a chronic disease a realistic strategy could be as follows:-

Week 1

Days 1 - 2   Psoric remedy e.g. *Psorinum* descending from 10M - 6C.

Days 3 - 7   Dyscrasia remedy e.g.*Hepar sulph* 30 in the morning.

Drainage remedy e.g. *Berberis* 30 in the middle of the day.

Indicated remedy in 30 potency in the evening.

Week 2   No remedies for at least one week.

Week 3

Days 1 - 2   Deep acting dyscrasia remedy e.g. *Radium bromide* or *Folliculinum* descended from 10M - 6C.

Days 3 - 7   Deeper dyscrasia remedy e.g.*Thuja* 30 in the morning.
Deeper drainage remedy e.g. *Kali phos* 30 in the middle of the day.
Indicated remedy in the 30 potency in the evening.

Weeks 4 and 5   No remedies for at least two weeks.

Week 6

Days 1 - 2   *Kali phos* - deeper drainage remedy descended from 10M - 6C.

Days 3 - 7   Dyscrasia remedy e.g. *Hepar sulph* 30 in the morning.
Kali Phos 30 in the middle of the day
Indicated remedy in 30 potency in the evening.

Weeks 7, 8 and 9 No remedies for at least three weeks.

Week 10

Day 1 - 2   Deeper drainage remedy e.g. *Causticum* descending from 10M - 6C.

Days 3 - 7   Dyscrasia remedy in 30 potency in the morning
Causticum 30 in the middle of the day
Indicated remedy 30 in the evening.

Weeks 11 - 14   No remedies for at least four weeks.

Then remedies given in descending order from 10M down, one potency each day, of *Psorinum* followed by *Hepar sulph* or other dyscrasia remedy, then the indicated remedy then *Tuberculinum*. Then either a break for two or three months before a possible repetition (if necessary) or to continue with deeper remedies, eg *Lycopodium* and *Silica*.

Appendix IV

The cases in this book show the use of a restricted number of remedies but also a variety of approaches with them We hope that we have given the homœopathic practitioner a strategy to help with those cases which have hitherto seemed resistant to treatment.

INDEX

S

T

U

V

W,X

Bibliography

Allen, J.H., *The Chronic Miasms*

Assilem, M.,*Folliculinum :Mist or Miasm*

Bhanja, K.C., *Constitution: Drug Pictures and Treatment* Calcutta National Homœopathic Laboratory, 1980.

Bianchi, I., *Allopathy, Homœopathy, Homotoxicology. An Outline.* Biological Therapy Vol. XI, No 3 1993.

Boericke, W.,*Materia Medica with Repertory* ,Philadelphia: Boericke and Tafel, 1976.

Burnett C., *New, Old and Forgotten Remedies*, 1906.

Chaitow, L., *Vaccination and Immunisation: Dangers, Delusions and Alternatives*, Saffron Walden, C.W. Daniel 1987.

Clarke, J., *Radium as an internal Remedy*, New Delhi, Jain Publishing Co., 1971.

Coulter, Catherine R., *Portraits of Homœopathic Medicines: Psychophysical Analyses of Selected Constitutional Types Vol. 1 and 2.* Washington D.C., Wehawken Book Company 1986 and 1988.

Dyson, R and Cole, J, *The Newsletter of the IBS Network,* Issue no 7, Autumn 1992.

Evans, J., *Spongia Tosta - A Study of its Signatures,* "The Homœopath", No. 61, The Society of Homœopaths, 1996.

Guernsey, H.N., *Keynotes to the Materia Medica.*

Hahnemann, S., *The Chronic Diseases: Their Peculiar Nature and The Homœopathic Cure,* New Delhi, Jain Publishing Co, 1978.

Hahnemann, S., *Organon of Medicine,* 6th Edition,Victor Gollancz Ltd, 1983

Hahnemann, S., *Materia Medica Pura,* New Delhi, Jain Publishing Co.

Hahnemann, S., and Dudgeon, *The Organon of Medicine,* New Delhi, Jain Publishing Co. 1970.

Hale, E.M., *New Remedies,* 3rd Edition.

Handley, R., *A Homœopathic Love Story,* Berkeley, North Atlantic Books, 1990.

Julian, O.A., *Materia Medica of New Homœopathic Remedies,* Beaconsfield Publishers Ltd, 1984.

Kent, J.T. *Lectures on Homœopathic Materia Medica,* New Delhi, Jain Publishing Co. 1972.

Kent J.T., *Clinical Cases,* New Delhi, Jain Publishing Co.

Kent, J.T., *Final General Repertory of the Homœopathic Materia Medica.* Revised, corrected, augmented and edited by Dr. Pierre Schmidt and Dr Diwan Harish Chand. Second Edition. New Delhi, National Homœopathic Pharmacy 1982.

Nash, E.B., *Leaders in Homœopathic Therapeutics,* Philadelphia, Boericke and Tafel, 1913.

Ongoing research of women in Massachusetts, New England, Journal of Medicine, October 1993.

Pall Mall Magazine, 17th October 1903

Phatak, S., *Materia Medica of Homœopathic Medicines,* Delhi, IBPS, 1977.

Sankaran, P., *The Clinical Relationship of Homœopathic Remedies,* Bombay, The Homœopathic Medical Publishers, 1984.